P9-ECW-108

i

A
CLINICAL GUIDE
FOR
CONTRACEPTION

A CLINICAL GUIDE FOR CONTRACEPTION

Leon Speroff, M.D.

Professor of Obstetrics and Gynecology
Oregon Health Sciences University
Portland, Oregon

Philip D. Darney, M.D., M.Sc.

Professor in Residence
Obstetrics, Gynecology and Reproductive Sciences
University of California, San Francisco
San Francisco, California

Illustration and Page Design
by Lisa Million, Portland, Oregon

Editor: *Michael Fisher*
Managing Editor: *Carol Eckhart*
Illustration and Page Design: *Lisa Million*
Production Coordinator: *Adele Boyd-Lanham*

Copyright (c) 1992
Williams & Wilkins
428 East Preston Street
Baltimore, Maryland 21202, USA

Accurate indications, adverse reactions, and dosage schedules for drugs are provided in this book, but it is possible that they may change. The reader is urged to review the package information data of the manufacturers of the medications mentioned.

Printed in the United States of America

First Edition 1992

Library of Congress Cataloging-in-Publication Data

Speroff, Leon, 1935.
    A clinical guide for contraception / Leon Speroff, Philip D. Darney.
        p. cm.
    Includes index.
    ISBN 0-683-07889-5
1. contraception. I. Darney, Philip D. II. Title.
(DNLM: 1. Contraception–methods. WP 630 S749c)
RG 136.S63 1992
613.9'4–dc20
DNLM / DLC
for Library of Congress

                                92–264
                                  CIP

Dedication

This book is dedicated to our children, one son and seven daughters. As Sherlock Holmes said: "You know my methods, use them!"

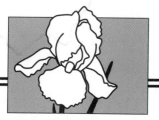

Preface

CONTRACEPTION, socially recognized and accepted only in the last 30 years, is both an essential and a complicated part of modern life. Contraception has separated sex from procreation and has provided couples greater control and enjoyment of their lives. It is a critical element in limiting population, thus preserving our planet's resources and maintaining quality of life for ourselves and our children. Contraception is both a personal and a social responsibility.

The above accomplishments could not be achieved by the simple contraceptive methods employed before the late 20th century. Greater effectiveness and ease of use required more complicated methods, associated with greater consequences to our health. Intensive study of these issues has yielded an enormous wealth of information, making an informed choice possible but not easy.

In this book, we have distilled and formulated the information essential for the intelligent use of contraception. The current state of knowledge and variety of contraceptive options allow clinicians and patients to select methods best suited to an individual's personal, social, and medical characteristics and requirements. But even now science is still sometimes inadequate, and medical judgments must be made without the comfort of scientific support. In these situations we have expressed our opinion, reflecting our knowledge and our clinical experience.

In addition to our children, we dedicate this book to all health care professionals who have assumed the social responsibility of assisting couples to use safe, effective contraception. We hope our text will help you and your patients.

Leon Speroff, M.D.
Portland, Oregon

Philip D. Darney, M.D.
San Francisco, California

Contents

1

Contraception in the U.S.A.

A S SOCIETIES become more affluent, fertility decreases. This decrease is in response to the use of contraception and abortion. During her reproductive lifespan, the average !Kung woman, a member of an African tribe of hunter-gatherers, experienced 15 years of lactational amenorrhea, 4 years of pregnancy, and only 48 menstrual cycles.[1] In contrast, a modern urban woman will experience 420 menstrual cycles. Contemporary women undergo earlier menarche and start having sexual intercourse earlier in their lives than in the past. Even though breastfeeding has increased in recent years, its duration is relatively brief, and its contribution to contraception in the developed world is trivial. Therefore, it is more difficult today to limit the size of a family unless some method of contraception is utilized.

More young women (under age 25) in America become pregnant than do their contemporaries in other Western countries.[2] The teenage pregnancy rates in 5 northern European countries and Canada range from 13 to 53% of the U.S. rate. The differences disappear almost completely after age 25. This is largely because American men and women after age 25 utilize surgical sterilization at a great rate.

It is obviously not true that young American women wish to have these higher pregnancy rates. American teenagers abort nearly half of their pregnancies, and this proportion is similar to that seen in other

2

countries. However, from ages 20–34, American women have the highest proportion of pregnancies aborted compared to other countries, indicating an unappreciated, but real, problem of unintended pregnancy existing beyond the teenage years. About half of all pregnancies in the U.S. are estimated to be unplanned and more than half of these are aborted.[2]

Another possible contribution to the problem of unintended pregnancy is the delay of marriage. Delaying marriage prolongs the period in which women are exposed to the risk of unintended pregnancy. This, however, cannot be documented as a major reason for the large differential between young adults in Europe and the U.S. The evidence available also indicates that a difference in sexual activity is not an important explanation. The major difference between American women and European women is that American women under age 25 are less likely to use any form of contraception.[2] Significantly the use of oral contraceptives (the main choice of younger women) is lower in the U.S. than in other countries.

Why are Americans different? The cultures in countries such as Canada and Britain are certainly very similar. A major difference must be attributed to the availability of contraception. In the rest of the world, contraceptive services can be obtained from more accessible resources and relatively inexpensively. In the rest of the world, contraception can be advertised on television. A further problem is the enormous diversity of people as well as the unequal distribution of income in the U.S. These factors influence the ability of our society to effectively provide education regarding sex and contraception, and to effectively make contraception services available.

The era of modern contraception dates from 1960 when oral contraception was first approved by the U.S. Food and Drug Administration, and intrauterine devices were re-introduced. For the first time, contraception did not have to be a part of the act of coitus. However, national family planning services and research were not funded by the U.S. Congress until 1970, and the last U.S. law prohibiting contraception was not reversed until 1973.

In 1966, a report from NASA placed our technological achievements into historical perspective.[3] Eight hundred lifespans can bridge more than 50,000 years. But of those 800 people:

- 650 spent their lives in caves,
- only the last 70 had a truly effective means of communication,
- only the last 6 saw the printed word,
- only the last 4 could measure time with precision,
- only the last 2 used an electric motor,
- and the majority of items which make up our current world were developed within the lifespan of the 800th person.

Contraception is not new; but its widespread development and application are new. It is in the latest tick of the Earth's timeclock, that safe control of fertility is now possible. This book is dedicated to that end. *This chapter will present an overview of the efficacy of contraceptive methods, a summary of contraceptive use in the U.S. and the world, and a brief look at the future.*

Efficacy of Contraception

A clinician's anecdotal experience is truly insufficient to provide the accurate information necessary for patient counseling. The clinician must be aware of the definitions and measurements used in assessing contraceptive efficacy, and must draw upon the talents of appropriate experts in this area to summarize the accurate and comparative failure rates for the various methods of contraception. A most helpful publication accomplishes these purposes and is highly recommended.[4]

Definition and Measurement

Contraceptive efficacy is generally assessed by measuring the number of unplanned pregnancies that occur during a specified period of exposure and use of a contraceptive method. The two methods which have been used to measure contraceptive efficacy are the Pearl index and life table analysis.

The Pearl Index. The Pearl index is defined as the number of failures per 100 woman-years of exposure. The denominator is the total months or cycles of exposure from the onset of a method until completion of the study, or an unintended pregnancy, or discontinuation of the method. The quotient is multiplied by 1200 if the denominator consists of months or by 1300 if the denominator consists of cycles.

4

With most methods of contraception, failure rates decline with duration of use. The Pearl index is usually based on a lengthy exposure (usually about a year) and therefore fails to accurately compare methods at various durations of exposure. This limitation is overcome by using the method of life table analysis.

Life Table Analysis. Life table analysis calculates a failure rate for each month of use. A cumulative failure rate can then compare methods for any specific length of exposure. Women who leave a study for any reason other than unintended pregnancy are removed from the analysis, contributing their exposure until the time of the exit.

Contraceptive failures do occur, and for many reasons. Thus "method effectivess" and "use effectiveness" have been used to designate efficacy with correct and incorrect use of a method. It is less confusing to simply compare the very best performance (the lowest expected failure rate) with the usual experience (typical failure rates) as noted in the table of failure rates during the first year of use. The lowest expected failure rates are determined in clinical trials, where the combination of highly motivated subjects and frequent support from the study personnel yields the best results.

Failure Rates During the First Year of Use, United States [5]

Method	Percent of Women with Pregnancy	
	Lowest Expected	Typical
No method	85.0%	85.0%
Combination Pill	0.1	3.0
Progestin only	0.5	3.0
IUDs		3.0
Progesterone IUD	2.0	<2.0
Copper T 380A	0.8	<1.0
Norplant	0.2	0.2
Female sterilization	0.2	0.4
Male sterilization	0.1	0.15
Depo-Provera	0.3	0.3
Spermicides	3.0	21.0
Periodic abstinence		20.0
Calendar	9.0	
Ovulation method	3.0	
Symptothermal	2.0	
Post–ovulation	1.0	
Withdrawal	4.0	18.0
Cervical cap	6.0	18.0
Sponge		
Parous women	9.0	28.0
Nulliparous women	6.0	18.0
Diaphragm and spermicides	6.0	18.0
Condom	2.0	12.0

6

Contraceptive Use in the U.S.

The National Survey of Family Growth is conducted every 5–6 years by the National Center for Health Statistics. Data are available from 1972, 1976, 1982, and 1988.[6,7] The sample is very large, and therefore, the estimates are very accurate.

Contraceptive Status and Method in Women 15–44 in 1988 [6,7]

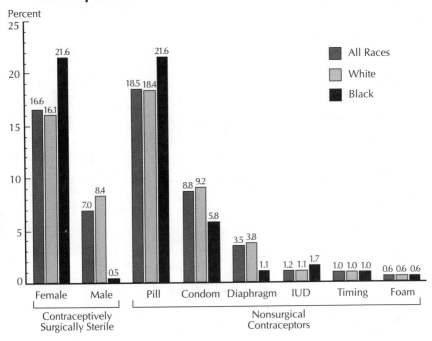

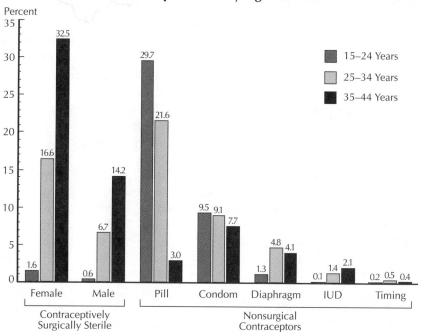

Contraceptive Use by Age in 1988 [6,7]

Percent

- 15–24 Years
- 25–34 Years
- 35–44 Years

Contraceptively Surgically Sterile
- Female: 1.6, 16.6, 32.5
- Male: 0.6, 6.7, 14.2

Nonsurgical Contraceptors
- Pill: 29.7, 21.6, 3.0
- Condom: 9.5, 9.1, 7.7
- Diaphragm: 1.3, 4.8, 4.1
- IUD: 0.1, 1.4, 2.1
- Timing: 0.2, 0.5, 0.4

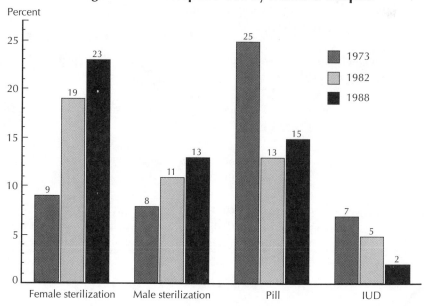

Changes in Contraceptive Use by Married Couples [6,7]

Percent

- 1973
- 1982
- 1988

- Female sterilization: 9, 19, 23
- Male sterilization: 8, 11, 13
- Pill: 25, 13, 15
- IUD: 7, 5, 2

8

The percent of married couples using sterilization as a method of contraception more than doubled from 1972 to 1988. In contrast, the percent of married couples using oral contraception declined sharply between 1973 and 1982. Recently, however, the use of oral contraception has increased, reaching a new high in 1991. About 10.7 million American women used oral contraceptives in 1988. Among never married women, oral contraception has been the leading method of birth control. Although condom use has not changed significantly among married couples, it did increase among never married women and is the second leading method.

In 1988, 60% of women, 15–44 years of age, were using contraception. Contraceptive sterilization was utilized by 24% of these women (the next leading method was oral contraception, 18.5%). The number of couples using the IUD decreased by two-thirds from 1981 to 1988, from 2.2 million to 0.7 million (7.1% to 2%). A total of 35 million of the 57.9 million women of reproductive age were using some method of contraception in 1988.

Of the 40% not using contraception, 7% were at risk of having an unintended pregnancy. Of the other 33%:

- 5%—sterilized for medical reasons,
- 1%—nonsurgically sterilized,
- 5%—pregnant,
- 4%—trying to get pregnant,
- 18%—not sexually active.

Thus, of those who are at risk of getting pregnant, 90% are using some method of contraception.

About 20 million women have one or more visits for contraceptive services per year in the U.S.

- 64% from a private doctor, group of doctors, or HMO,
- 36% from a public clinic.

A difference by race in contraceptive visits (greater among blacks) is present only until age 20. By ages 35–44, over half of women or their husbands are surgically sterile, either for contraceptive or medical reasons.

6

For added insight, it is useful to compare the choices of American women with Swedish women.[8,9] Swedish women mostly use the pill, condoms or the IUD; 95% of those exposed to risk of pregnancy practice contraception. Older Swedish women are more likely to rely on the IUD or barrier methods.

Contraceptive Choices in Sweden and the U.S. [8,9]

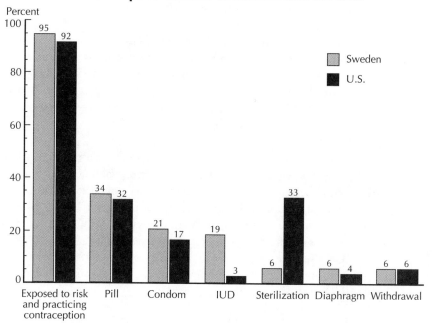

Abortion in the U.S.A. The number of abortions performed in the United States has remained relatively unchanged since 1980, approximately 1.6 million per year.[10] About 29% of pregnancies not ending in miscarriage or stillbirth are terminated by abortion. The proportion of abortions performed in hospitals has steadily declined, reaching 10% in 1988. The proportion handled by specialized abortion clinics increased to 86% by 1988, while the percentage of abortions performed by physicians in their own offices has remained low, about 3–5% of all abortions. More than 50% of abortions are obtained by women younger than 25, with the rate peaking at ages 18–19, and 83% are unmarried.[11]

10

U.S. Characteristics. Malcolm Potts has reviewed the history, development, and future of birth control in the United States.[12] He points out that while there was rapid progress in the 1960s and 1970s, over the last 10–15 years, "everything began to fall apart." Today U.S. women have fewer birth control choices than women in other industrialized nations, and contraception is more expensive. He concludes that these are the reasons that American women have higher rates of unintended childbirth and abortion compared to women in other industrialized nations.

Another contrast is oral contraceptive use among older married women. In the Netherlands, for example, it is nearly twice as high in 20–29 year old women as among comparable U.S. women, and among women over 35, the level in the Netherlands is nearly 10 times that in the U.S. Conversely, the total abortion rate in the U.S. is almost 3 times that of Dutch women.

It is not surprising that U.S. couples have made up for the lack of contraceptive choices by greater reliance on voluntary sterilization. With the current trend, it wouldn't be long before 3 out of 4 American couples choose sterilization within 15 to 20 years of their last wanted birth. During the years of maximal fertility, oral contraceptives are the most common method peaking at age 20–24. Most IUD users are concentrated between ages 25 and 40, and even here there are differences: four times as many French women over 40 use IUDs compared to American women.

Among 30–44 year olds, therefore, sterilization is the most utilized method of family planning. Between 1973 and 1982, oral contraception and sterilization changed places as the most popular contraceptive method among married women over the age of 25. The rate of sterilization among American women over 35 is about the same compared to Great Britain and the Netherlands, but under the age of 30 it is 50% higher in American women.

In young women, the frequency of sexual intercourse is associated with the choice of contraceptive.[13] Young people who are very active sexually prefer oral contraception because it is perceived as very effective and allows sex to be worry free. As concern with AIDS grows, a more favorable attitude towards the condom is emerging.

Worldwide Use of Contraception

The world population is expected to stabilize at between 10 and 11 billion by the year 2100.[14] Approximately 95% of the growth will occur in developing countries, so that by 2100, 13% of the population will live in developed countries, a decrease from the current 25%.

World Population

1 billion—achieved in 1800–1850
2 billion—achieved in 1930
3 billion—achieved in 1960
4 billion—achieved in 1976
5 billion—achieved in 1987

Throughout the world, 45% of married women of reproductive age practice contraception. However, there is significant variation from area to area; for example, 69% in East Asia, but only 11% in Africa. Female sterilization and the IUD are most popular in developing countries, while oral contraceptives and condoms are most popular in developed countries. Of the 400 million women of reproductive age, less than 60 million (15%) are using oral contraceptives, and more than half live in the U.S., Brazil, France, and Germany.

Number of Couples Using Birth Control Methods in 1986 [15]

Method	China	Rest of Developing World	Developed World	Total World
Female sterilization	53 mill.	45 mill.	15 mill.	113 mill.
IUDs	59	13	11	83
Oral contraceptives	9	28	27	64
Condoms	5	12	28	45
Male sterilization	17	18	8	43
Other methods	3	8	13	24

The 76% of the world's population living in developing countries accounts for:

- 85% of all births,
- 95% of all infant and childhood deaths,
- 99% of all maternal deaths.

The problem in the developing world is self-evident. The ability to regulate fertility has a significant impact on infant, child, and maternal mortality and morbidity. A pregnant woman has a 200 times greater chance of dying living in a developing country rather than in a developed country.[14]

The Impact of Use and Non-Use

Inadequate access to contraception is associated with a high abortion rate. Effective contraceptive use largely, although not totally, replaces the resort to abortion.[16] The combination of restrictive abortion laws and the lack of safe abortion services continues to make unsafe abortion a major cause of morbidity and mortality throughout the world. Both safe and unsafe abortions can be minimized by maximizing contraceptive services. However, the need for safe abortion services will persist. Contraceptive failures account for about half of the 1.5 million annual induced abortions in the U.S.

In the U.S. in the late 1980s, $1 spent on public funding for family planning saved an average of $4.40 spent on medical, welfare, and nutritional services.[17] The investment in family planning leads to short-term reductions in expenditures on maternal and child health services, and after 5 years, a reduction in costs for education budgets.

Cutting back on publicly funded family planning services impacts largely on poor women, increasing the number of unintended births and abortions. In California, there is an average of $7.70 saved for every $1 spent to provide contraceptive services.[18] This estimate is higher than the national estimate because the income ceiling for eligibility is higher in California.

There is a gap between the low levels of unintentional pregnancy that can be achieved and the actual levels being obtained, most of which is in couples using reversible contraception. A major thrust, in addition to providing services, must include education and counseling of couples in effective contraception.

STDs and Contraception

The interaction between clinician and patient for the purpose of contraception provides an opportunity to control sexually transmitted diseases (STDs). The modification of unsafe sexual practices reduces the risk of unplanned pregnancy and the risk of infections of the reproductive tract. A patient visit for contraception is an excellent time for STD screening; if an infection is symptomatic, it should be diagnosed and treated during the same visit in which contraception is requested. A positive history for STDs should trigger both screening for asymptomatic infections and counseling for safer sexual practices. Attention should be given to the contraceptive methods which have the greatest influence on the risk of STDs.

Contraception and Litigation

Clinicians are concerned about the prospect of bad outcomes associated with contraceptive use leading to litigation. Multimillion dollar verdicts and settlements in favor of plantiffs who have used products as innocent as spermicides capture national attention. Actually, these events are very unusual compared to the widespread use of contraception.

The best way to avoid litigation is good patient communication. Patients who sue usually claim there were contraindications or risks that were not conveyed by the clinician. The best way to influence litigation is to keep good records. Good clinician's records are the most formidable weapon for the defense. Documentation is vital, but it is useless without thorough history taking. Good records and good history taking put the responsibility on the patient's honesty in response to the clinician.

> *Document that the risks and benefits of all methods were discussed.*
> *Document a plan for follow-up.*
> *Document all interactions with the patient, including phone calls.*

14

The Future

From 1970 to 1986, the number of births in women over 30 quadrupled. As more and more couples defer pregnancy until later in life, the use of sterilization under age 35 will decline, and the need for reversible contraception will increase. In 1988, 75% of pill users were under age 30. Only 5% of women 35–44 used oral contraception, compared to 38% under age 25. These numbers will change only if clinicians and patients understand and accept that low dose oral contraception is safe for healthy, nonsmoking older women.

The percent of married couples using sterilization as a method of contraception more than doubled from 1972 to 1988. In contrast, the percent of married couples using oral contraception declined sharply between 1973 and 1982.[7] Nevertheless, the need for reversible contraception in women over the age of 30 is growing, not diminishing.

The highest ever number of births in the U.S. occurred between 1947 and 1965—the post World War II baby boom. Women born in this period won't be through reaching their 45th birthday until around 2010. For approximately a 20 year period, therefore, there will be an unprecedented number of women in the later child-bearing years. It is estimated that the number of women ages 35–49 will increase 61% between 1982 and 1995. The proportion of births accounted for by this group of women will increase by about 72%, from 5% in 1982 to 8.6% in 2000.[19] This group of women is not only increasing in number, but it is changing its fertility pattern.

The deferment of marriage is a significant change in our society. In 1960, 28% of women 20–24 were single; in 1985, 58.5%. In 1960, 10% of women 25–29 were single; in 1985, 26%. But only 16% of the decline in the total fertility rate is accounted for by the increase in the average age at first marriage. Eighty-three percent of the decline in total fertility rate is accounted for by changes in marital fertility rates. In other words postponement of pregnancy in marriage is the more significant change.[20] This combination of increasing numbers, deferment of marriage, and postponement of pregnancy in marriage is responsible for the fact that we will be seeing more and more older women who will need reversible contraception. In short, there will be longer duration of use in younger women and greater use in older women. Indeed, this pattern of use was being observed by 1990.

Change in Female Demographics 1985–2000 [21]

Age	1985	1990	1995	2000	% Change 1985–2000
15–24	19.5 mill.	17.4 mill.	16.7 mill.	17.7 mill.	-9.2%
25–29	10.9	10.6	9.3	8.6	-21.1
30–34	10.0	11.0	10.8	9.4	-6.0
35–44	16.2	19.1	21.1	21.9	+35.2
Total 15–44	56.6	58.1	57.9	57.6	+1.8

One solution to the problem of a restricted number of choices for American women is to develop new methods. However, experts are pessimistic when it comes to looking forward to new methods. There are many obstacles to the development of new methods, including the attitudes of the American public (Besides America's traditionally conservative, religion-oriented views towards sex and family, polarization is produced by responses evoked by specific issues such as sterilization and abortion.), the funding available for research, the time and cost required to meet federal regulations, and the problems of product liability.[22]

Fortunately clinicians and patients have recognized that low dose oral contraception is very safe for healthy, nonsmoking older women. However, as the above statistics indicate, its use is still not sufficient to meet the need. Besides fulfilling a need, this population of women has a series of benefits to be derived from oral contraception that tilt the risk/benefit ratio to the positive side. The following benefits are especially pertinent for older women:

Effective contraception.
- less need for therapeutic abortion.
- less need for surgical sterilization.

Less endometrial cancer.
Less ovarian cancer.
Less benign breast disease.
Fewer ovarian cysts.
Fewer uterine fibroids.
Fewer ectopic pregnancies.
More regular menses.
- less flow.
- less dysmenorrhea.
- less anemia.

Less salpingitis.
Less rheumatoid arthritis.
Increased bone density.
Probably less endometriosis.
Possibly protection against atherosclerosis.

The growing need for reversible contraception would also be served by increased utilization of the IUD. After several years of use, efficacy with the IUD is similar to that of oral contraceptives. The decline in IUD use in the U.S. is in direct contrast to the experience in the rest of the world, a complicated response to publicity and litigation. An increased risk of pelvic infection with contemporary IUDs in use is limited to the act of insertion and the transportation of pathogens to the upper genital tract. This risk is effectively minimized by careful screening with pre-insertion cultures and the use of good technique. A return to IUD use by American couples is both warranted and desirable.

Contraceptive advice is a component of good preventive health care. The approach is a key. This is an era of informed choice by the patient. Patients deserve to know the facts and need help in dealing with the state of the art and the uncertainty. But there is no doubt that patients, especially young patients, are influenced in their choice by their clinician's advice and attitude. While the role of a clinician is to provide the education necessary for the patient to make proper choices, one should not lose sight of the powerful influence exerted by the clinician in the choices ultimately made.

If one attempts to sum the impact of the benefits of contraception on public health, as some have done with models focusing on hospital admissions, there is no doubt that the benefits outweigh the risks. The impact can be measured in terms of both morbidity and mortality.

AND DON'T FORGET THE IMPACT ON A COUPLE'S SOCIAL AND PERSONAL LIFE: A GREATER FREEDOM TO MAKE DECISIONS.

But the impact on public health is of little concern during the private clinician-patient interchange in the medical office. Here personal risk is paramount, and compliance with effective contraception requires accurate information.

In our view, the attitude of the clinician is a crucial influence on the ultimate patient take home message. In the 70s we approached the patient with great emphasis on risk. In the 90s the approach should be different, highlighting the benefits and the greater safety of appropriate contraception.

The challenge for the next 20 years is to do as Sherlock Holmes said: "You know my methods, use them."[23] A stable global population of about 8–10 billion is possible. Without better contraceptive education and services, global population could reach 15 billion before stabilization.

18

References

1. Djerassi C, *The Politics of Contraception, Vol I. The Present,* Stanford Alumni Association, Stanford, California, 1979.

2. Westoff CF, Unintended pregnancy in America and abroad, Fam Plann Persp 20:254, 1988.

3. Lesher RL, Howick GJ, Assessing technology transfer, NASA Report SP-50671, 1966.

4. Trussell J, Hatcher RA, Cates W Jr, Stewart FH, Kost K, A guide to interpreting contraceptive efficacy studies, Obstet Gynecol 76:558, 1990.

5. Trussell J, Hatcher RA, Cates W Jr, Stewart FH, Kost K, Contraceptive failure in the United States: An update, Stud Fam Plann 21:51, 1990.

6. Mosher WD, Pratt WF, Contraceptive use in the United States, 1973–88, Advance data from vital and health statistics; No. 182, National Center for Health Statistics, Hyattsville, Maryland, 1990.

7. Mosher WD, Use of family planning services in the United States: 1982 and 1988, Advance data from vital and health statistics, No. 184, National Center for Health Statistics, Hyattsville, Maryland, 1990.

8. Forrest JD, Fordyce RR, U.S. women's contraceptive attitudes and practice: How have they changed in the 1980s? Fam Plann Persp 20:112, 1988.

9. Riphagen FE, von Schoultz B, Contraception in Sweden, Contraception 39:633, 1989.

10. Henshaw SK, Van Vort J, Abortion services in the United States, 1987 and 1988, Fam Plann Persp 22:102, 1990.

11. Henshaw SK, Induced abortion: A world review, 1990, Fam Plann Persp 22:76, 1990.

12. Potts M, Birth control methods in the United States, Fam Plann Persp 20:288, 1988.

13. Glor JE, Severy LJ, Frequency of intercourse and contraceptive choice, J Biosoc Sci 22:231, 1990.

14. Diczfalusy E, The worldwide use of steroidal contraception, Int J Fertil 34 (Supplement):56, 1989.

15. Population Crisis Committee, Access to birth control: A world assessment, Population Briefing Paper No. 19, Washington, DC, 1986.

16. Potts M, Rosenfield A, The fifth freedom revisited: I. Background and existing programs, Lancet 336:1227, 1990.

17. Forrest JD, Singh S, Public-sector savings resulting from expenditures for contraceptive services, Fam Plann Persp 22:6, 1990.

18. Forrest JD, Singh S, The impact of public-sector expenditures for contraceptive services in California, Fam Plann Persp 22:161, 1990.

19. Spencer G, Projections of the population of the United States, by age, sex, and race: 1983–2080. Current Population Reports—Population Estimates and Projections, US Department of Commerce, May 1984, Series P-25, No. 952.

20. Westoff CF, Fertility in the United States, Science 234:554, 1986.

21. Spencer G, Projections of the population of the United States by age, sex and race: 1988–2080, Current Population Reports 1989, Series P-25, No. 1018, GPO, Washington, DC, 1989.

22. Mastroianni L Jr, Donaldson PJ, Kane TT, editors, *Developing New Contraceptives: Obstacles and Opportunities,* National Academy Press, Washington, DC, 1990.

23. Doyle AC, *The Sign of Four.*

2

Oral Contraception

CONTRACEPTION is commonly viewed as a modern event, a recent development in human history. On the contrary, efforts to limit reproduction predate our ability to write about it. It is only oral contraception with synthetic sex steroids that is recent.

History

It wasn't until the early 1900s, that inhibition of ovulation was observed to be linked to pregnancy and the corpus luteum. Ludwig Haberlandt, professor of physiology at the University of Innsbruck, Austria, was the first to demonstrate that ovarian extracts given orally could prevent fertility (in mice).[1,2] In the 1920s, Haberlandt and a Viennese gynecologist, Otfried Otto Fellner, were administering steroid extracts to a variety of animals and reporting the inhibition of fertility. By 1931, Haberlandt was proposing the administration of hormones for birth control. An extract was produced, named Infecundin, ready to be used, but Haberlandt's early death in 1932, at age 47, brought an end to this effort. Fellner disappeared after the fall of Austria to Hitler.

The concept was annunciated by Haberlandt, but steroid chemistry wasn't ready. The extraction and isolation of a few milligrams of the sex steroids required starting points measured in gallons of urine, or thousands of pounds of organs. Edward Doisy processed 80,000 sow

21

ovaries to produce 12 mg of estradiol.

Russell Marker. The supply problem was solved by an eccentric chemist, Russell E. Marker, who completed his thesis, but not his course work, for his Ph.D. After leaving school, Marker worked with the Ethyl Gasoline Corporation, and in 1926, developed the process of octane rating, based on the discovery that knocking in gasoline was due to hydrocarbons with an uneven number of carbons.

From 1927 to 1935, Marker worked at the Rockefeller Institute, publishing a total of 32 papers on configuration and optical rotation as a method of identifying compounds. In 1935, he moved to Pennsylvania State University where he trained himself in steroid chemistry and became interested in solving the problem of producing abundant and cheap amounts of progesterone. At that time it required the ovaries from 2,500 pregnant pigs to produce 1 mg of progesterone. In 1939, Marker became convinced that the solution to the problem of obtaining large quantities of steroid hormones was to find plants (in the family that includes the lily, the agave, and the yam) which contained sufficient amounts of sapogenin, a plant steroid which could be used as a starting point for steroid hormone synthesis. This conviction was strengthened with his discovery that a species of *Trillium*, known locally as Beth's root, was collected in North Carolina and used in the preparation of Lydia Pinkham's Compound, popular at the time to relieve menstrual troubles. The active ingredient in Beth's root was diosgenin, a plant steroid.

Marker organized extensive botanical expeditions in the Southwest and Mexico, sending home more than 100,000 pounds of material. In 1942, he collected the roots of the Mexican yam, and back in Pennsylvania, he worked out the degradation of diosgenin to progesterone. United States pharmaceutical companies refused to back Marker, and even the University refused, despite Marker's urging, to patent the process.

In 1943, Marker resigned from Pennsylvania State University and went to Mexico where he collected the roots of *Dioscorea mexicana*, ten tons worth! In an old pottery shed in Mexico City, in two months, he prepared several pounds of progesterone (worth $600,000). This progesterone gained him entry to Hormone Laboratories in Mexico City. The 2 partners in Hormone Laboratories and Marker formed a company which they called Syntex. The price of progesterone fell from $200 to $2 a gram.

In 1947, true to his eccentric nature, Marker had a falling out with his partners and sold his share of the company, retiring to Pennsylvania to devote the rest of his life to making replicas of antique works in silver. However, he took his knowhow with him. Fortunately for Syntex, he had published a scientific description of his process, and there still was no patent on his discoveries. Syntex recruited George Rosenkranz, a Hungarian immigrant living in Cuba, to reinstitute the commercial manufacture of progesterone (and testosterone) from Mexican yams, a task which took him 2 years.

Carl Djerassi. In 1949, it was discovered that cortisone relieved arthritis, and the race was on to develop an easy and cheap method to synthesize cortisone. Carl Djerassi joined Syntex to work on this synthesis using the Mexican yam plant steroid diosgenin as the starting point. This was quickly achieved (in 1951), but soon after, an even better method of cortisone production was discovered at Upjohn, using microbiologic fermentation. This latter method used progesterone as the starting point, and therefore, Syntex found itself as the key supplier to other companies for this important process, at the rate of 10 tons of progesterone per year and a price of 48 cents per gram.

Djerassi and other Syntex chemists then turned their attention to the sex steroids. They discovered that the removal of the 19 carbon from yam-derived progesterone increased the progestational activity of the molecule. Ethisterone had been available for a dozen years, and the Syntex chemists reasoned that removal of the 19 carbon would increase the progestational potency of this orally active compound. In 1951, norethindrone was synthesized; the patent for this drug is the only patent for a drug listed in the National Inventor's Hall of Fame in Washington. Two years later, G.D. Searle & Company filed a patent for norethynodrel.

Gregory Pincus. Gregory Pincus of the Worcester Foundation for Experimental Biology in Massachusetts had been studying mammalian fertilization for many years.[3] He attributed his shift of interest to contraception to a visit from Margaret Sanger in 1951. Sanger, president of the International Planned Parenthood Federation, provided a research grant of $2,100 for animal research, and pointed out that Pincus' animal experiments suggested a method of oral contraception for women.

Both the Syntex and Searle compounds were tested by Gregory Pincus, John Rock, and colleagues in animals in 1953–1954, and in the first human trial, in 1956, with the help of Edris Rice-Wray, a pioneer in family planning who was working at the time in Puerto Rico. The initial progestin products were contaminated with about 1% mestranol. In the amounts being used, this added up to 50–500 micrograms of mestranol, a sufficient amount of estrogen to inhibit ovulation by itself. When efforts to lower the estrogen content yielded breakthrough bleeding, it was decided to retain the estrogen for cycle control, thus establishing the principle of the combined estrogen-progestin oral contraceptive.

Pincus, a long-time consultant to Searle, picked the Searle compound for extended use. Syntex, a wholesale drug supplier, was without marketing experience or organization. Pincus with great effort convinced Searle that the commercial potential of an oral contraceptive warranted the risk of possible negative public reaction. By the time Syntex had secured arrangements with Ortho for a sales outlet, Searle marketed Enovid in 1960 (150 µg mestranol and 9.85 mg norethynodrel). Ortho-Novum using norethindrone from Syntex appeared in 1962. Wyeth Laboratories introduced norgestrel in 1968, the same year in which the first reliable prospective studies were initiated. It was not until the late 1970s that a dose-response relationship between problems and the amount of steroids in the pill was appreciated. As a result, health care providers and patients, over the years, have been confronted by a bewildering array of different products and formulations. The solution to this clinical dilemma is relatively straightforward: use the lowest doses that provide effective contraception.

Pharmacology of Steroid Contraception

Basic Chemistry

All steroid hormones are of basically similar structure with relatively minor chemical differences leading to striking alterations in biochemical activity. The basic structure is the perhydrocyclopentanephenanthrene molecule. It is composed of three 6-carbon rings and one 5-carbon ring. One ring is benzene, two rings naphthalene, and three rings phenanthrene; add a cyclopentane (5-carbon ring) and you have the perhydrocyclopentanephenanthrene structure of the steroid nucleus.

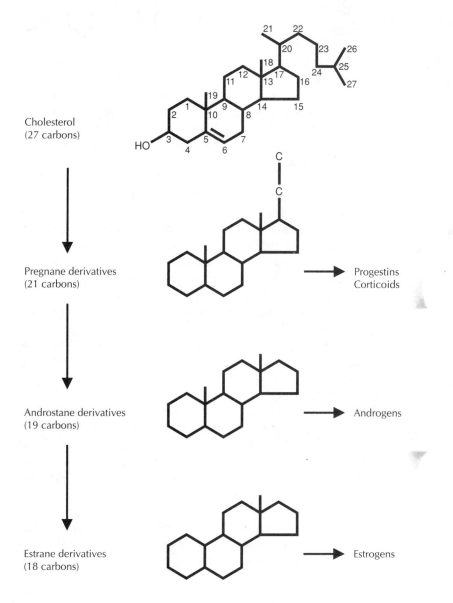

Cholesterol
(27 carbons)

Pregnane derivatives
(21 carbons) → Progestins Corticoids

Androstane derivatives
(19 carbons) → Androgens

Estrane derivatives
(18 carbons) → Estrogens

The sex steroids are divided into 3 main groups according to the number of carbon atoms they possess. The 21-carbon series includes the corticoids and the progestins and the basic structure is the *pregnane* nucleus. The 19-carbon series includes all the androgens and is based on the *androstane* nucleus, whereas the estrogens are 18-carbon steroids based on the *estrane* nucleus.

There are 6 centers of asymmetry on the basic ring structure, and there are 64 possible isomers. Almost all naturally occurring and active steroids are nearly flat, and substituents below and above the plane of the ring are designated alpha (α) (dotted line) and beta (β)(solid line), respectively. Changes in the position of only one substituent can lead to inactive isomers. For example, 17-epitestosterone is considerably weaker than testosterone, the only difference being a hydroxyl group in the α position at C-17 rather than in the β position.

The convention of naming steroids uses the number of carbon atoms to designate the basic name (e.g. pregnane, androstane, or estrane). The basic name is preceded by numbers which indicate the position of double bonds and the name is altered as follows to indicate 1, 2, or 3 double bonds: -ene, -diene, and -triene. Following the basic name, hydroxyl groups are indicated by the number of the carbon attachment, and 1, 2, or 3 hydroxyl groups are designated -ol, -diol, or -triol. Ketone groups are listed last with numbers of carbon attachments, and 1, 2, or 3 groups designated -one, -dione, or -trione. Special designations include: dehydro, elimination of 2 hydrogens; deoxy, elimination of oxygen; nor, elimination of carbon; delta or Δ, location of double bond.

Lipids and Cholesterol. Cholesterol is the basic building block in steroidogenesis. All steroid-producing organs except the placenta can synthesize cholesterol from acetate. Progestins, androgens, and estrogens, therefore, can be synthesized in situ in the various ovarian tissue compartments from the 2-carbon acetate molecule via cholesterol as the common steroid precursor. However, the major resource is blood cholesterol which enters the ovarian cells and can be inserted into the biosynthetic pathway, or stored in esterified form for later use. The cellular entry of cholesterol is mediated via a cell membrane receptor for low-density lipoprotein (LDL), the bloodstream carrier for cholesterol.

Estrone
1,3,5(10)-Estratriene-3β-ol-17-one

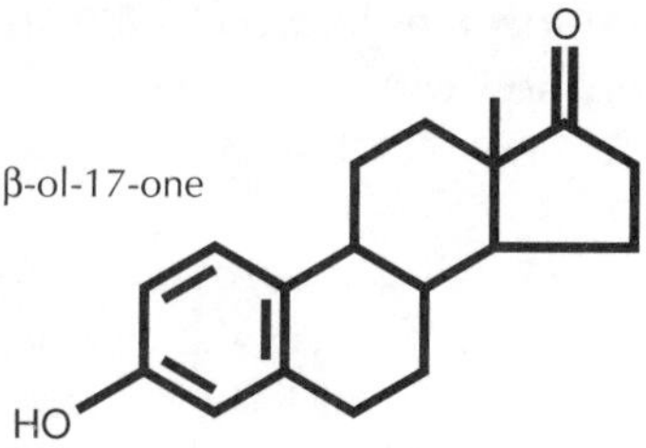

Testosterone
4-Androstene-17β-ol-3-one

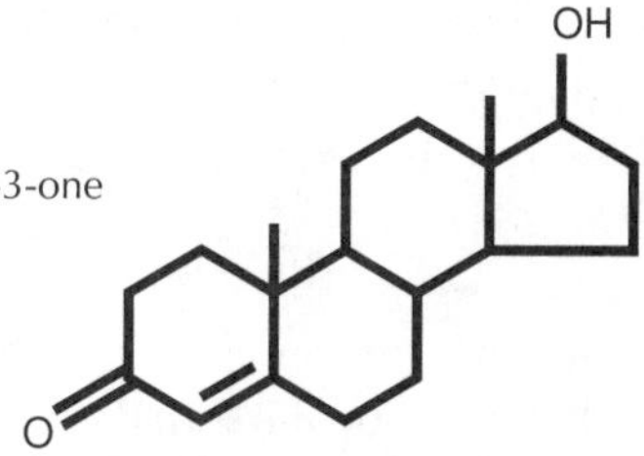

CH₃

Progesterone
4-Pregnene-3,20-dione

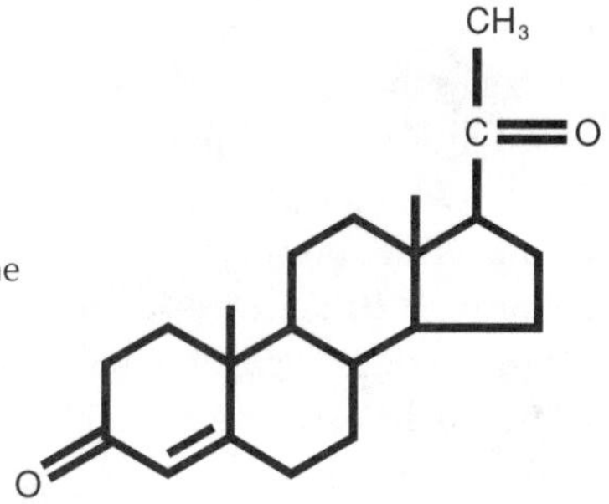

Lipoproteins are large molecules that facilitate the transport of nonpolar fats in a polar solvent, the blood plasma. There are 5 major categories of lipoproteins according to their charge and density (flotation during ultracentrifugation). They are derived from each other in the following cascade of decreasing size and increasing density:

Chylomicrons. Large, cholesterol (10%) and triglyceride (90%) carrying particles formed in the intestine after a fatty meal.

Very Low-Density Lipoproteins (VLDL). Also carry cholesterol, but mostly triglyceride; more dense than chylomicrons.

Intermediate-Density Lipoproteins (IDL). Formed (for a transient existence) with the removal of some of the triglyceride from the interior of VLDL particles.

Low-Density Lipoproteins (LDL). The end products of VLDL catabolism, formed after further removal of triglyceride leaving approximately 50% cholesterol; the major carriers (2/3) of cholesterol in the plasma and thus a strong relationship exists between elevated LDL levels and cardiovascular disease.

High-Density Lipoproteins (HDL). The smallest and most dense of the lipoproteins with the highest protein and phospholipid content; HDL levels are inversely associated with atherosclerosis (high levels are protective).

The lipoproteins contain 4 ingredients: 1) cholesterol in two forms: free cholesterol on the surface of the spherical lipoprotein molecule, and esterified cholesterol in the molecule's interior; 2) triglyceride in the interior of the sphere; 3) phospholipid and 4) protein: electrically charged substances on the surface of the sphere and responsible for miscibility with plasma and water. The surface proteins, called *apoproteins*, constitute the sites which bind to the lipoprotein receptor molecules on the cell surfaces. The principal protein of LDL is apoprotein B, and apoprotein A-I is the principal apoprotein of HDL. These protein moieties of the lipoprotein particles are strongly related to the risk of cardiovascular disease, and genetic abnormalities in their synthesis or structure can result in atherogenic conditions.

The liver synthesizes a high molecular weight protein (apoprotein B-100) which is secreted as a component of VLDL. VLDL are composed of triglyceride, cholesterol, and smaller proteins (apoprotein E and apoprotein C). VLDL transport triglyceride in the blood and are metabolized in tissues by the action of the enzyme lipoprotein lipase, leaving remnant forms which are cleared by the liver. In this way, cholesterol and triglyceride are transported, metabolized, processed, and excreted. When this system becomes saturated (e.g. by a high fat diet) remnant particles remaining in the plasma lose their triglyceride leaving predominantly cholesterol-containing particles which are further degraded to LDL. The apoprotein B-100 remains on LDL, while the smaller proteins are removed.

HDL are composed of proteins (primarily apoprotein A-I and apoprotein A-II) synthesized in the liver and intestine, and which combine with lipids removed from other lipoproteins and tissue. HDL of increasing size and cholesterol content are known as HDL_3, HDL_{2a}, and HDL_{2b}. HDL returns cholesterol to the liver, so-called reverse cholesterol transport.

Thus the level of apoprotein A-I is a marker of reverse transport efficiency, while the level of apoprotein B is correlated with LDL levels and accumulation of LDL particles. The biologic effect of apo A-II is not yet understood. In the liver the enzyme hepatic lipase degrades lipid components and is strongly influenced by hormones.

The lipoproteins are a major reason for the disparity in arteriosclerosis risk between men and women. Throughout adulthood, the blood HDL-cholesterol level is about 10 mg/dl higher in women, and this difference continues through the postmenopausal years. Total and LDL-cholesterol levels are lower in premenopausal women than in men, but after menopause they rise rapidly.

LDL is removed from the blood by organ (mainly liver) receptors which recognize one of the surface apoproteins. The liver is the favored site for this process because it contains the largest number of LDL receptors as well as a unique high affinity receptor for one of the apoproteins, apoprotein E. The lipoprotein bound to the cell membrane receptor is internalized and degradated. When these LDL receptors are saturated or deficient, LDL is taken up by "scavenger" cells (most likely derived from macrophages) in other tissues, most notably the arterial intima. Thus these cells can become the nidus for atherosclerotic plaques.

The protective nature of HDL is due to its ability to pick up free cholesterol from cells or other circulating lipoproteins. Thus HDL converts lipid-rich scavenger cells back to their low-lipid state, and carries the excess cholesterol to sites (mainly liver) where it can be metabolized.

For good cardiovascular health, the blood concentration of cholesterol must be kept low and its escape from the bloodstream into arterial intima must be prevented. The problem of cholesterol transport is solved by esterifying the cholesterol and packaging the ester within the cores of plasma lipoproteins. The delivery of cholesterol to cells is in turn solved by lipoprotein receptors. After binding the lipoprotein with its package of esterified cholesterol, the complex is delivered into the cell by receptor-mediated endocytosis, where the lysosomes liberate cholesterol for use by the cell.

Major protection against atherosclerosis depends upon the high affinity of the receptor for LDL and the ability of the receptor to recycle multiple times, thus allowing large amounts of cholesterol to be delivered while maintaining a healthy low blood level of LDL. Cells can control their uptake of cholesterol by increasing or decreasing the number of LDL receptors according to the intracellular cholesterol levels.

There are 3 important clinical points:

1. Atherosclerotic disease is related to increased LDL and decreased HDL-cholesterol concentrations.
2. Lowering LDL levels and raising HDL levels can reduce the incidence of atherosclerotic disease.
3. Atherosclerosis is not a disease limited to aging people. It begins in early childhood, and its manifestation later in life can be influenced by health care behavior during younger years.

The following actions are associated with estrogens (the opposite occurs with progestins):

- Synthesis of apoprotein B-100 is increased.
- Synthesis of triglyceride is increased.
- Hepatic lipase activity is suppressed (increases HDL).
- Synthesis of apoprotein A-I is increased (increases HDL).
- Clearance (catabolism) of LDL is increased.

The Estrogen Component

Estradiol is the most potent natural estrogen, and is the major estrogen secreted by the ovaries. The major obstacle to the use of sex steroids for contraception was inactivity of the compounds when given orally. A major breakthrough occurred in 1938 when it was discovered that the addition of an ethinyl group at the 17 position made estradiol orally active. Ethinyl estradiol is a very potent oral estrogen and is one of the two forms of estrogen in every oral contraceptive. The other estrogen is the 3-methyl ether of ethinyl estradiol, mestranol.

Ethinyl estradiol   Mestranol

Mestranol and ethinyl estradiol are different from natural estradiol and must be regarded as pharmacologic drugs. Animal studies have suggested that mestranol is weaker than ethinyl estradiol, because mestranol must first be converted to ethinyl estradiol in the body. Indeed, mestranol will not bind to the cellular estrogen receptor. Therefore, unconjugated ethinyl estradiol is the active estrogen in the blood for both mestranol and ethinyl estradiol. In the human body, differences in potency between ethinyl estradiol and mestranol do not appear to be significant, certainly not as great as indicated by assays in rodents. This is now a minor point since all of the low dose oral contraceptives contain ethinyl estradiol.

The metabolism of ethinyl estradiol (particularly as reflected in blood levels) varies significantly from individual to individual, and from one population to another.[4] There is even a range of variability at different sampling times within the same individual. Therefore, it is not surprising that the same dose can cause side effects in one individual and none in another.

The estrogen content (dosage) of the pill is of major clinical impor-tance. Thrombosis is one of the most serious side effects of the pill, playing a key role in the increased risk of death from a variety of circulatory problems. This side effect is related to estrogen, and it is dose related. Therefore, the dose of estrogen is a critical issue in selecting an oral contraceptive.

The Progestin Component

The discovery of ethinyl substitution and oral potency led (at the end of the 1930s) to the preparation of ethisterone, an orally active derivative of testosterone. In 1951, it was demonstrated that removal of the 19 carbon from ethisterone to form norethindrone did not destroy the oral activity, and most importantly, it changed the major hormonal effect from that of an androgen to that of a progestational agent. Accordingly, the progestational derivatives of testosterone were designated as 19-nortestosterones (denoting the missing 19 carbon). The androgenic properties of these compounds, however, were not totally eliminated and minimal anabolic and androgenic potential remains within the structure.

Testosterone   Ethisterone

Ethisterone   Norethindrone

The "impurity" of 19-nortestosterones, i.e. androgenic as well as progestational effects, was further complicated in the past by a belief that they were metabolized within the body to estrogenic compounds. This question was restudied, and it was argued that the previous evidence for metabolism to estrogenic compounds was due to an artifact in the laboratory analysis. More recent studies indicate that norethindrone can be converted to ethinyl estradiol, however the rate of this conversion is so low, that insignificant amounts of ethinyl estradiol can be found in the circulation or urine following the administration of the commonly used doses of norethindrone.[5] Any estrogenic activity, therefore, would have to be due to a direct effect. In animal and human studies, however, only norethindrone, norethynodrel, and ethynodiol diacetate have estrogen activity, and it is very slight due to weak binding to the estrogen receptor.[6] Clinically, androgenic and estrogenic activities of the progestin component are, therefore, insignificant due to the low dosage in the new oral contraceptives. As with the estrogen component, serious side effects have been related to the high doses of progestins used in old formulations, not the particular progestin, and routine use of oral contraceptives should now be limited to the low dose products.

33

The norethindrone family contains the following 19-nortestosterone progestins: norethindrone, norethynodrel, norethindrone acetate, ethynodiol diacetate, lynestrenol, norgestrel, norgestimate, desogestrel, and gestodene.

Most of the progestins closely related to norethindrone are converted to the parent compound. Thus the activity of norethynodrel, norethindrone acetate, ethynodiol diacetate, and lynestrenol is due to rapid conversion to norethindrone.

Norgestrel is a racemic equal mixture of the dextrorotatory enantiomer and the levorotatory enantiomer. These enantiomers are mirror images of each other and rotate the plane of polarized light in opposite directions. The dextrorotatory form is known as d-norgestrel, and the levorotatory form is l-norgestrel (known as levonorgestrel). Levonorgestrel is the active isomer of norgestrel.

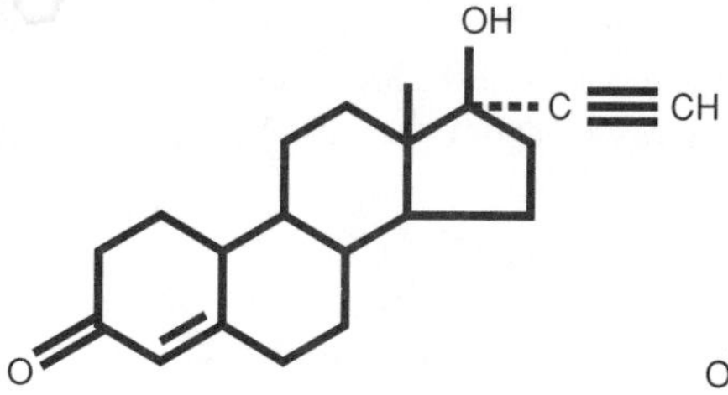

Norethindrone

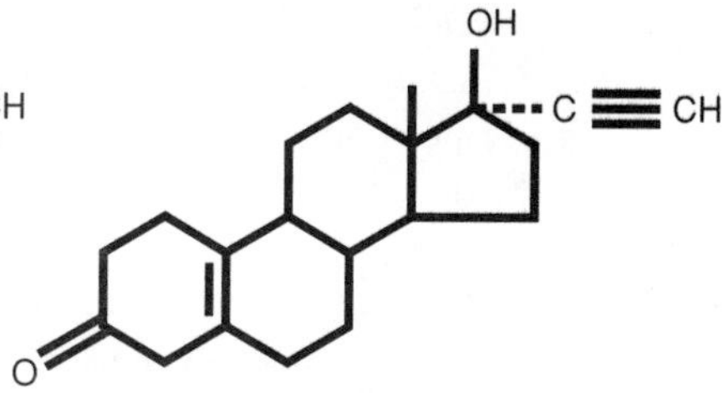

Norethynodrel

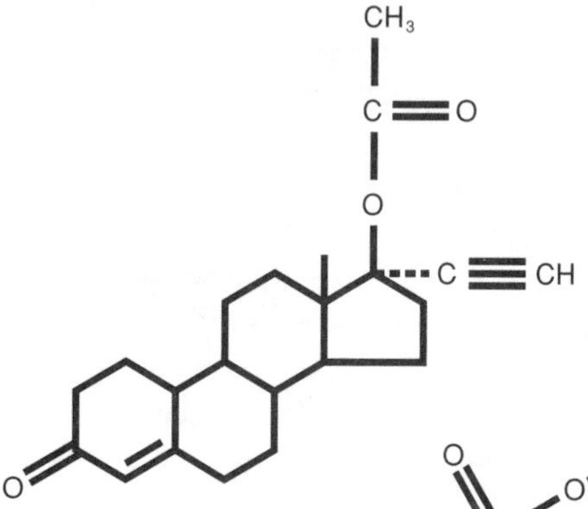

Norethindrone acetate

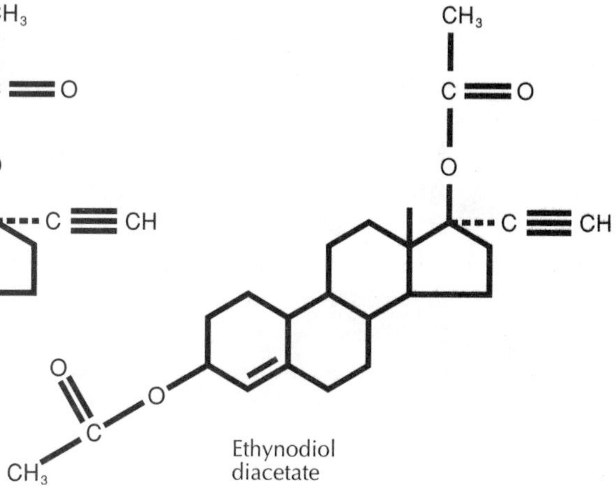

Ethynodiol diacetate

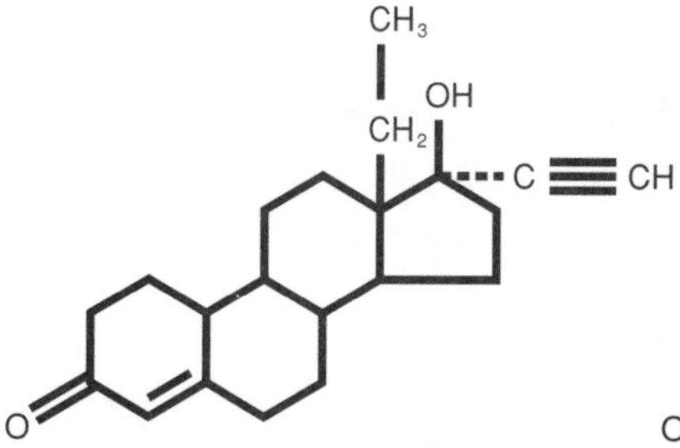

Levonorgestrel

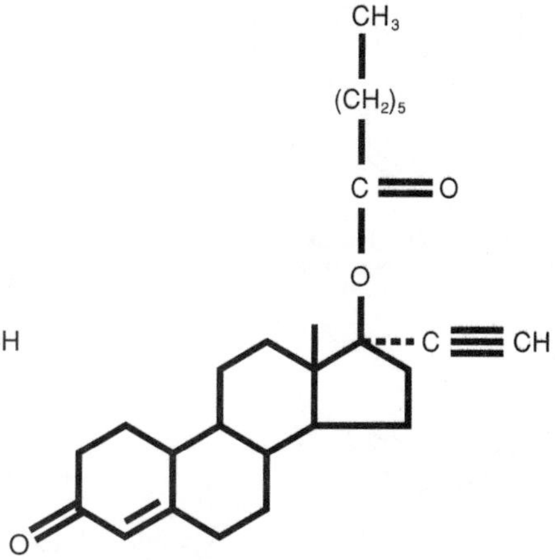

Norethindrone enanthate

Desogestrel undergoes two metabolic steps before the progestational activity is expressed in its active metabolite, 3-keto-desogestrel. This metabolite differs from levonorgestrel only by a methylene group in the 11 position.

Gestodene differs from levonorgestrel by the presence of a double bond between carbons 15 and 16, thus it is delta 15 gestodene. It is metabolized into many derivatives with progestational activity, but not levonorgestrel.

Several metabolites contribute to the activity of norgestimate, including 17-deacetylated norgestimate, 3-keto norgestimate, and levonorgestrel.

A second group of progestins became available for use when it was discovered that acetylation of the 17-hydroxy group of 17-hydroxyprogesterone produced an orally active but weak progestin. An addition at the 6 position is necessary to give sufficient progestational strength for human use, probably by inhibiting metabolism. Derivatives of progesterone with substituents at the 17 and 6 positions include the widely used medroxyprogesterone acetate.

17α-Hydroxyprogesterone   17-Acetoxy progesterone

Medroxyprogesterone acetate
(Provera)

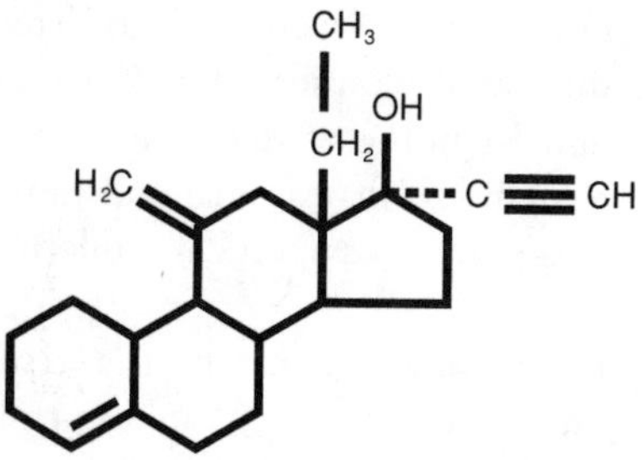

Desogestrel

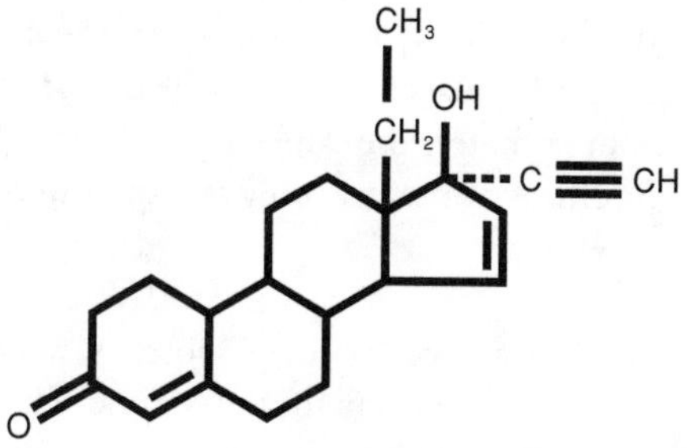

Gestodene

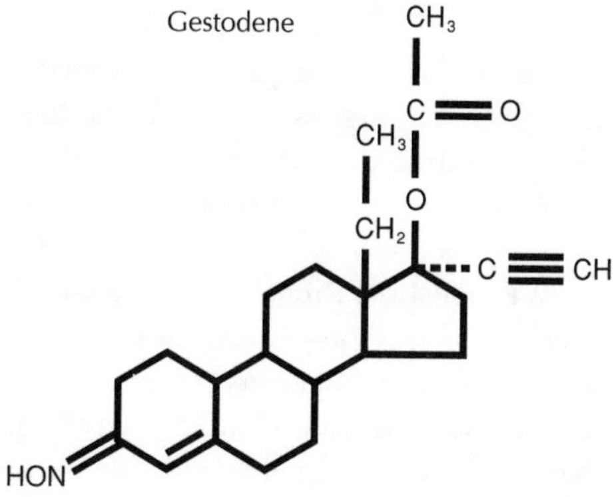

Norgestimate

Potency. For many years, clinicians, scientists, medical writers, and even the pharmaceutical industry have attempted to assign potency values to the various progestational components of oral contraceptives. An accurate assessment, however, has been difficult to achieve for many reasons. Progestins act on numerous target organs (e.g. the uterus, the mammary glands, and the liver), and potency varies depending upon the target organ and endpoint being studied. In the past, animal assays, such as the Clauberg test and the rat ventral prostate assay, were used to determine progestin potency. While these were considered acceptable methods at the time, a better understanding of steroid hormone action and metabolism, and a recognition that animal and human responses differ, have led to greater reliance upon data collected from human studies.

Historically, this has been a confusing issue as publications and experts used potency ranking to provide clinical advice. There is absolutely no need for confusion. Oral contraceptive progestin potency is no longer a consideration when it comes to prescribing oral contraception, because the potency of the various progestins has been accounted for by appropriate adjustments of dose. In other words, the biologic effect (in this case the clinical effect) of the various progestational components in current low dose oral contraceptives is approximately the same. The potency of a drug does not determine its efficacy or safety, only the amount of a drug required to achieve an effect.

Clinical advice based on potency ranking is an artificial exercise which has not stood the test of time. There is no clinical evidence that a particular progestin is better or worse in terms of particular side effects or clinical responses. Thus oral contraceptives should be judged by their clinical characteristics: efficacy, side effects, risks, and benefits. Our progress in lowering the doses of the steroids contained in oral contraceptives has yielded products with little serious differences. Potency is no longer an important clinical issue.

New Progestins. Probably the greatest influence on the effort which yielded the new progestins was the belief throughout the 80s that androgenic metabolic effects were important, especially in terms of cardiovascular disease. (Cardiovascular side effects are now known to be due to a dose-related stimulation of thrombosis by estrogen.) In the search to find compounds which minimize androgenic effects, however, the pharmaceutical companies succeeded.

The new progestins include desogestrel, gestodene, and norgestimate. With the combined products containing the new progestins, the changes in the coagulation system are very similar to those with the current low dose formulations. A slight prothrombotic effect is characterized by increased levels of fibrinopeptide A which is balanced by antithrombin III and protein C. Thus any coagulation tendency is counteracted. The protime and the activated partial thromboplastin time measure the overall activity of the coagulation pathways—there is no significant increase in these measurements with the new formulations.

All progestins derived from 19-nortestosterone have the potential to decrease glucose tolerance and increase insulin resistance. The impact of the current low dose formulations is very minimal, and the impact of the new progestins is negligible. Most changes are not statistically significant, and when they are, they are so subtle as to be of no clinical significance. For example, there are no changes in hemoglobin A1c.

The new progestins, because of their reduced androgenicity, predictably do not adversely affect the cholesterol-lipoprotein profile. Indeed, the estrogen-progestin balance of combined oral contraceptives containing one of the new progestins may even promote favorable lipid changes. Thus, the new formulations have the potential to offer protection against cardiovascular disease, an important consideration as we enter an era of women using oral contraceptives for longer durations and later in life. But one must be cautious regarding the clinical significance of subtle changes, and it will be a long time before epidemiologic data on this issue are available.

New Formulations

The latest development in oral contraceptive technology is the multiphasic preparation which alters the dosage of both the estrogen and progestin components periodically throughout the pill-taking schedule. The future will bring even more products and different formulations. The aim of these new formulations is to alter steroid levels in an effort to achieve lesser metabolic effects and minimize the occurrence of breakthrough bleeding and amenorrhea, while maintaining efficacy. We are probably at or very near the lowest dose levels which can be achieved without sacrificing efficacy. Metabolic studies with the multiphasic preparations indicate no differences or slight improvements over the metabolic effects of low dose monophasic products. Clinicians and patients are urged to choose a new multiphasic preparation or to use the low dose (less than 50 µg estrogen) monophasic pills. The use of higher dose pills should be discontinued, and all women on higher dose pills should be changed to low dose preparations. Stepping down the dose can be safely accomplished with absolutely no decrease in efficacy. The therapeutic principle remains: utilize the pills which give effective contraception and the greatest margin of safety.

Mechanism of Action

The combination pill, consisting of the estrogen and progestin components, is given daily for 3 out of every 4 weeks. The combination pill prevents ovulation by inhibiting gonadotropin secretion via an effect on both pituitary and hypothalamic centers. The progestational agent in the pill primarily suppresses luteinizing hormone (LH) secretion (and thus prevents ovulation), while the estrogenic agent suppresses follicle-stimulating hormone (FSH) secretion (and thus prevents the selection and emergence of a dominant follicle). Therefore, the estrogenic component significantly contributes to the contraceptive efficacy. However, even if follicular growth and development were not sufficiently inhibited, the progestational component would prevent the surge-like release of LH necessary for ovulation.

The estrogen in the pill serves two other purposes. It provides stability to the endometrium so that irregular shedding and unwanted breakthrough bleeding can be minimized; and the presence of estrogen is required to potentiate the action of the progestational agents. The latter function of estrogen has allowed reduction of the progestational dose in the pill. The mechanism for this action is probably estrogen's effect in increasing the concentration of intracellular progestational receptors. Therefore, a certain pharmacologic level of estrogen is necessary to maintain the potency of the combination pill.

Since the effect of a progestational agent will always take precedence over estrogen (unless the dose of estrogen is increased many, many fold), the endometrium, cervical mucus, and perhaps tubal function reflect progestational stimulation. The progestin in the combination pill produces an endometrium which is not receptive to ovum implantation, a decidualized bed with exhausted and atrophied glands. The cervical mucus becomes thick and impervious to sperm transport. It is possible that progestational influences on secretion and peristalsis within the Fallopian tubes provide additional contraceptive effects.

Efficacy

With this variety of contraceptive actions, it is hard to understand how the omission of a pill or two can result in a pregnancy. Indeed, careful review of failures suggests that pregnancies usually occur because initiation of the next cycle is delayed allowing escape from ovarian suppression. Strict adherence to 7 pill-free days is critical in

Failure Rates During the First Year of Use, United States [7]

Method	Percent of Women with Pregnancy	
	Lowest Expected	Typical
No method	85.0%	85.0%
Combination Pill	0.1	3.0
Progestin only	0.5	3.0
IUDs		3.0
Progesterone IUD	2.0	<2.0
Copper T 380A	0.8	<1.0
Norplant	0.2	0.2
Female sterilization	0.2	0.4
Male sterilization	0.1	0.15
Depo-Provera	0.3	0.3
Spermicides	3.0	21.0
Periodic abstinence		20.0
Calendar	9.0	
Ovulation method	3.0	
Symptothermal	2.0	
Post–ovulation	1.0	
Withdrawal	4.0	18.0
Cervical cap	6.0	18.0
Sponge		
Parous women	9.0	28.0
Nulliparous women	6.0	18.0
Diaphragm and spermicides	6.0	18.0
Condom	2.0	12.0

41

order to obtain reliable, effective contraception. For this reason, the 28 day pill package, incorporating 7 pills which do not contain steroids, is a very useful aid to assure adherence to the necessary schedule.

The contraceptive effectiveness of the multiphasic formulations are unequivocally comparable to low dose (less than 50 µg estrogen) and higher dose monophasic combination birth control pills. While carefully monitored studies with motivated subjects achieve an annual failure rate of 0.1%, typical usage is associated with a 3.0% failure rate during the first year of use.[7] Efficacy decreases significantly when the estrogen component is removed, and only a small dose of the progestin is administered (the progestin-only minipills).

Metabolic Effects of Oral Contraception

Cardiovascular Disease

A major problem for clinicians is that we and our patients live in the present, but we must use data from the past. Nowhere is this more true than in the area of oral contraception where the data are derived from older pills of higher dosage while current clinical practice utilizes lower dose pills and new formulations.

Much of what we knew and taught for several decades was derived from two major British prospective cohort studies.[8-15] The Royal College of General Practitioners (RCGP) study began in 1968 with 23,000 pill users matched with 23,000 non-users. The Oxford/Family Planning Association (OFPA) study involves 17,032 women. A third cohort study, the American Walnut Creek study enrolled 16,638 women between 1968 and 1972.[16]

The reports from these studies and from American case-control studies heavily influenced clinicians and patients. The following observations were derived from these reports over a period of approximately 10 years:

1. Venous thrombosis is a dose-related effect of estrogen, limited to current users only, with a disappearance of the risk by 4–6 weeks after discontinuing oral contraception as the coagulation factors rapidly return to normal. The risk of deep venous thrombosis in the leg is 4 times greater in higher dose oral contraceptive users

than nonusers, and that of superficial thrombosis in the leg, 2 times greater. There is no evidence that varicose veins have any influence on deep thrombosis associated with oral contraceptive use.

2. The risk of myocardial infarction is increased in women over age 35, and consideration of other risk factors (hypertension, hypercholesterolemia, cigarette smoking, obesity, and diabetes mellitus) indicated that oral contraceptives acted synergistically with them, rather than additively.[17-20] In the 1983 RCGP report, only older (over age 35) smokers currently using oral contraceptives had a statistically significant increased risk of ischemic heart disease compared to controls.[12]

3. The British data also indicated a relationship between progestin doses and the risk of cardiovascular disease, *but it is important to note that the British studies found an increased risk only with progestin doses no longer utilized.*[21,22] Because older high dose pills were used by older women in these studies, the results are further confounded by their inclusion of women at higher risk because of age.

4. Clinical reports were consistent with an association between the use of higher dose oral contraceptives and neurovascular accidents in otherwise healthy young women. According to retrospective studies, oral contraceptive use increased the risk of thrombotic stroke 3-fold, and that of hemorrhagic stroke, 2-fold.[23] The RCGP 1983 report and the 1984 OFPA report indicated that the increased risk of stroke was approximately doubled.[12,15]

We cannot emphasize strongly enough that the above conclusions were derived from patients and pills that no longer commonly, if at all, encounter each other! In response to the above reports, clinicians became more strict in their screening of patients and prescribing of oral contraception, at the same time as lower dose formulations (less than 50 μg of estrogen) came to dominate the market.

Two forces, therefore, were at work simultaneously to bring greater safety to women utilizing oral contraception: the use of lower dose pills and the avoidance of oral contraception by high risk patients. For these reasons, the Walnut Creek study and the Puget Sound study in the United States did not find an increased risk of myocardial infarction with the use of oral contraceptives.[16,24] When healthy patients on low dose pills were studied (Walnut Creek by its study population and Puget Sound by design), no significant association between stroke and oral contraceptives was observed. A report from OFPA emphasized that after 9100 woman-years of use, not a single patient on the low dose pills had suffered a stroke.[15]

Analyses of vital statistics data in the United States and in 21 countries in Europe, Asia, and North America failed to reveal the high levels of death from cardiovascular diseases associated with oral contraceptive use which the early British data suggested would occur.[25,26] In December, 1980, the Walnut Creek study reported no significant differences in mortality rates between ever and never users of oral contraceptives.[16] A short time later, the RCGP and OFPA updated their ongoing studies and supported the favorable conclusions of Walnut Creek.[11,14] The important observations reported in 1981 included the following:

1. Duration of oral contraceptive use had no effect on mortality when age was controlled.
2. The effect of age was less than previously thought. The increased morality in users was concentrated in smokers over the age of 35. Users under the age of 35 (smokers and nonsmokers) had minimally increased mortality risks that could have arisen by chance.
3. For women age 35 to 44, the major risk is in smokers, and nonsmokers without risk factors for vascular disease can expect the benefits of oral contraceptive use to outweigh the risks.
4. Deaths from cerebral vascular disease and heart disease accounted for most of the increased mortality, with pulmonary embolism accounting for only 10%.

Both the RCGP and OFPA studies indicated, therefore, that women under the age of 35, regardless of smoking status, are at no significantly increased risk of death when taking oral contraceptives. Mortality data using the new low dose pills support this favorable outlook.[27] In 54,971 woman-years of oral contraceptive use in the Seattle area, there were no cardiovascular deaths among users compared with 11 cardiovascular deaths in the nonuser group.[24]

The Coagulation System and Oral Contraception. The goal of the clotting mechanism is to produce thrombin, which converts fibrinogen to a fibrin clot. Thrombin is generated from prothrombin by factor Xa in the presence of factor V, calcium, and phospholipids. The vitamin K-dependent factors include factors VII, IX, and X, as well as prothrombin. Antithrombin III is one of the body's natural anticoagulants, an irreversible inhibitor of thrombin and factors IXa, Xa, and XIa. Protein C and protein S are two other major inhibitors of coagulation and are also vitamin K-dependent. Deficiencies of antithrombin III, protein C, and protein S are inherited in an autosomal dominant pattern.

Tissue plasminogen activator (t-PA) is produced by endothelial cells and released when a clot forms. Both t-PA and plasminogen bind to the fibrin clot. The t-PA converts the plasminogen to plasmin which lyses the clot by degrading the fibrin.

The minimal risk of thrombosis associated with oral contraceptive use does not justify the cost of routine screening for deficiencies in the coagulation system. If a patient develops a thrombotic complication while taking oral contraceptives, an evaluation to search for an underlying abnormality in the coagulation system is warranted (measurement of antithrombin III, protein C, protein S, activated partial thromboplastin time, fibrinogen, and plasminogen).

Swedish and RCGP reports indicated that women who use 50 μg estrogen pills have a higher incidence of venous thrombosis than those who use lower dose pills.[21,28] A review of the massive Medicaid data in the state of Michigan confirms the fact that the risk of venous thrombosis is increased at the 50 μg dose.[29] It is still unknown whether a risk of venous thrombosis persists at the lower doses. Studies of the blood coagulation system have concluded that both monophasic and multiphasic low dose oral contraceptives are associated with homeostasis. Slight increases in thrombin formation are offset by increased fibrinolytic activity.[30–34]

Today, the rare young woman on oral contraception who has a thrombotic episode probably represents someone with an underlying clotting problem, an individual who shows an extreme response to oral contraceptives, or an individual with an unknown lesion of a vessel wall or an unknown local disturbance of circulation.

There is no evidence of an increase in risk of cardiovascular disease among past users of oral contraception.[35-37] In the Nurses' Health Study, impressive for its accurate and long-term follow-up of a very large cohort of women, there is no evidence of a trend toward an increase in risk with duration of use, and there is an immediate decline in risk to baseline after cessation of oral contraception.[35] (Remember, these data are derived from older days, different pills, and less effective screening). Why is this important? Because it points to a short-term mechanism. Part of the concern for a possible lingering effect of oral contraceptive use is based upon a presumed adverse impact on the atherosclerotic process which would then be added to the effect of aging, and thus manifested later in life. *Instead, the findings are consistent with the contention that cardiovascular disease due to oral contraception is secondary to acute effects, specifically estrogen-induced thrombosis, a dose-related event.*

Lipoproteins and Oral Contraception. The balance of estrogen and progestin potency in a given oral contraceptive formulation can influence cardiovascular risk by its overall effect on lipoprotein levels. Oral contraceptives with relatively high doses of progestins (doses not used in today's low dose formulations) do produce unfavorable lipoprotein levels.[38] The levonorgestrel triphasic exerts no significant changes on HDL-cholesterol, LDL-cholesterol, apoprotein B, and no change or an increase in apoprotein A, while the levonorgestrel monophasic combination (with a higher dose of levonorgestrel) has a tendency to increase LDL-cholesterol and apoprotein B, and to decrease HDL-cholesterol and apoprotein A.[39-42] The monophasic desogestrel pill has a favorable effect on the lipoprotein profile, while the triphasic gestodene pill produces only slight changes, which are beneficial alterations in the LDL/HDL and apoprotein B/apoprotein A ratios.[39-42] Like the triphasic levonorgestrel pills, norethindrone multiphasic pills have no significant impact on the lipoprotein profile over 6–12 months.[43] *In summary, studies of low dose formulations indicate that the adverse effects of progestins are limited to the fixed dose combination with levonorgestrel, a dose of levonorgestrel that exceeds that in the multiphasic formulation.*

During the past few years we have been subjected to considerable marketing hype in regards to the importance of the impact of oral contraceptives on the cholesterol-lipoprotein profile. If indeed certain oral contraceptives had a negative impact on the lipoprotein profile, one would expect to find evidence of atherosclerosis as a cause of an increase in subsequent cardiovascular disease. There is no such evidence. Thus the mechanism of the cardiovascular complications is undoubtedly a short-term acute mechanism, thrombosis (an estrogen-related effect).

This conclusion is reinforced by angiographic and autopsy studies. Young women with myocardial infarctions who have used oral contraceptives have less diffuse atherosclerosis than non-users.[44,45] Indeed, a case-control study indicated that the risk of myocardial infarction in patients taking levonorgestrel-containing formulations is the same as that experienced with pills containing other progestins.[46]

These conclusions have significant bearing on the choice of a contraceptive. It certainly is a good pharmacologic principle to utilize a medication with least impact on normal physiology. However, if this impact is so subtle that it is clinically insignificant, then this issue is of relatively little importance when it comes to selecting an oral contraceptive. Current evidence suggests there is no advantage or disadvantage associated with any of the current low-dose formulations in regards to cardiovascular disease. However, it seems prudent to avoid the higher doses of progestins such as 150–250 µg of levonorgestrel, The low doses of levonorgestrel (such as in the multiphasic formulations) do not have an adverse impact on the lipid profile.

An important study in monkeys has indicated a protective action of estrogen against atherosclerosis, but by a mechanism independent of the cholesterol-lipoprotein profile. Oral administration of a combination of estrogen and progestin to monkeys fed a high cholesterol, atherogenic diet decreased the extent of coronary atherosclerosis despite a reduction in HDL-cholesterol levels.[47–49] In somewhat similar experiments, estrogen treatment markedly prevented arterial lesion development in rabbits.[50–52] In considering the impact of progestational agents, lowering of HDL is not necessarily atherogenic if accompanied by a significant estrogen impact. These animal studies help explain why older, higher dose combinations which had an adverse impact on the lipoprotein profile did not increase subsequent cardiovascular disease. The estrogen component provided protection through a direct effect on vessel walls. Perhaps the low dose combinations will even be associated with a favorable impact on the risk of cardiovascular disease.

The first epidemiologic data on this issue derived from low dose oral contraception come from Finland and England. Preliminary analysis of cardiovascular deaths among women under 40 years of age in Finland indicates a statistically significant reduction in low dose oral contraceptive users in the relative risk of myocardial infarction (RR = 0.2) and stroke (RR = 0.7).[53] In England, studies from the RCGP and OFPA now report no increased risk in *current* users, as previously indicated in studies of higher dose pills.[37,54] The numbers are still small, however, and the reports still cannot establish whether the reduced risk is due to lower doses or better screening.

There currently is no statistically significant evidence that any specific oral contraceptives containing different progestational components in low doses have a major advantage or disadvantage when side effects are compared. Furthermore, it should be recognized that the clinical relevance of the lipid modifications remains to be substantiated by epidemiologic data. It is appropriate to question the clinical and biological significance of the reported changes because the great majority of the changes have still been within the physiologic ranges for age and sex.

Conclusion. The low dose pills are safer than the pills previously used. The overall risk is minimal in healthy women who do not smoke, and under the age of 35 the synergistic effect of smoking appears to be negligible. Only smokers 35 and older have a significantly increased risk of dying from circulatory diseases. Vascular events in younger, healthy women (if they still occur at lower doses) may now be confined to outliers, patients with underlying subtle defects which are unmasked or enhanced by oral contraceptive use.

Hypertension

Oral contraceptive-induced hypertension was observed in approximately 5% of users of higher dose pills.[8] More recent evidence indicates that small increases in blood pressure can be observed even with 30 μg estrogen, monophasic pills,[55-57] however an increased incidence of clinically significant hypertension has not been reported. No significant clinical changes in blood pressure have been noted with any of the multiphasic formulations. It is possible for an occasional patient to experience an idiosyncratic reaction and develop hypertension, therefore, an annual assessment of blood pressure is still an important element of clinical surveillance, even when low dose oral contraceptives are used.

The mechanism for an effect on blood pressure is thought to involve the renin angiotensin system. The most consistent finding is a marked increase in plasma angiotensinogen, the renin substrate, up to 8 times normal values (on higher dose pills). In nearly all women, excessive vasoconstriction is prevented by a compensatory decrease in plasma renin concentration. If hypertension does develop, the renin-angiotensinogen changes take 3–6 months to disappear after stopping combined oral contraception.

Variables such as previous toxemia of pregnancy or previous renal disease do not predict whether a woman will develop hypertension on oral contraception.[58] Likewise, women who have developed hypertension on oral contraception are not more predisposed to develop toxemia of pregnancy.

One must also consider the effects of oral contraceptives in patients with pre-existing hypertension or cardiac disease. Data from the RCGP continue to indicate that the presence of hypertension in oral contraceptive users increases the risk of myocardial infarction.[37] It is still unknown whether this risk is present with low dose pills. In our view, with medical control of the blood pressure and close follow-up, the patient and her clinician may choose low dose oral contraception. Close follow-up is also indicated in women with a history of pre-existing renal disease or a strong family history of hypertension or cardiovascular disease. It seems prudent to suggest that patients with marginal cardiac reserve should utilize other means of contraception. Significant increases in cardiac output and plasma volume have been recorded with oral contraceptive use (higher dose pills), probably a result of fluid retention.

Carbohydrate Metabolism

With the older high dose oral contraceptives, an impaired glucose tolerance test was present in many women. In these women, plasma levels of insulin as well as the blood sugar were elevated. Generally the effect of oral contraception is to produce an increase in peripheral resistance to insulin action. Most women can meet this challenge by increasing insulin secretion, and there is no change in the glucose tolerance test.

Carbohydrate metabolism is affected mainly by the progestin component of the pill. The derangement of carbohydrate metabolism may also be affected by estrogen influences on lipid metabolism, hepatic enzymes, and elevation of unbound cortisol. The glucose intolerance is dose-related, and once again effects are less with the low dose formulations. *Insulin and glucose changes with low dose monophasic and multiphasic oral contraceptives are so minimal, that it is now believed that they are of no clinical significance.*[59-61] This includes long-term evaluation with hemoglobin A1c. The one exception is the claim that the levonorgestrel monophasic has an excessively negative impact.

The observed changes in studies of oral contraception and carbohydrate metabolism are in the nondiabetic range. In order to measure differences, investigators have resorted to analysis by measuring the area under the curve for glucose and insulin responses during glucose tolerance tests. A highly regarded cross-sectional study utilizing this technique reported that even lower dose formulations have detectable effects on insulin resistance.[62] The reason this is important is that it is argued that hyperinsulinemia due to insulin resistance is now a recognized contributor to cardiovascular disease. However, there are several critical questions that remain unanswered. Can the results from a cross-sectional study be duplicated in a study of sufficient size with patients serving as their own controls? Is a statistically significant hyperinsulinemia detected in a study clinically meaningful?

Because long-term, follow-up studies of large populations have failed to detect any increase in the incidence of diabetes mellitus or impaired glucose tolerance (even in past and current users of high dose pills),[63,64] the concern now focuses on the slight impairment as a potential risk for cardiovascular disease. If slight hyperinsulinemia were meaningful, wouldn't you expect to see evidence of an increase in cardiovascular disease in past users who took oral contraceptives when doses were higher? As we have emphasized before, there is no such evidence. The data strongly indicate that the changes in lipids and carbohydrate metabolism that have been measured are not clinically meaningful.

It can be stated definitively that oral contraceptive use does not produce an increase in diabetes mellitus.[64,65] The hyperglycemia associated with oral contraception is not deleterious and is completely reversible. Even women who have risk factors for diabetes in their history do not seem to be affected.

There is some controversy regarding the response of women with previous gestational diabetes mellitus. Kung et al. report higher plasma insulin levels and a deterioration of glucose tolerance after 6 months of the levonorgestrel triphasic.[65] On the other hand, Skouby et al. reported no effect over 6 months on either glucose tolerance or lipids.[66,67] It should be noted that the abnormal results reported by Kung et al. are due to abnormal data in 4 of 11 women. In a larger study of women with recent gestational diabetes, no significant impact could be demonstrated over 6–13 months comparing a low dose monophasic and a multiphasic to a control group.[68] We can expect a high percentage of women with previous gestational diabetes to develop overt diabetes and associated vascular complications. Until overt diabetes develops, we believe it is appropriate for these patients to use low dose oral contraception.

In clinical practice, it may, at times, be necessary to prescribe oral contraception for the overt diabetic. The effect on insulin requirement is neither consistent nor predictable, but one would expect little, if any, change with low dose pills. According to the epidemiologic data, the use of oral contraceptives increases the risk of thrombosis in women with insulin-dependent diabetes mellitus; therefore, women with diabetes should be encouraged to use other forms of contraception. However this effect in women under age 35 who are otherwise healthy is probably very minimal with low dose oral contraception, and reliable protection against pregnancy is a benefit for these patients that outweighs the small risk.

The Liver

The liver is affected in more ways and with more regularity and intensity by the sex steroids than any other extragenital organ. Estrogen influences the synthesis of hepatic DNA and RNA, hepatic cell enzymes, serum enzymes formed in the liver, and plasma proteins. Estrogenic hormones also affect hepatic lipid and lipoprotein formation, the intermediary metabolism of carbohydrates, and intracellular enzyme activity.

The active transport of biliary components is impaired by estrogens as well as some progestins. The mechanism is unclear, but cholestatic jaundice and pruritus were occasional complications of higher dose oral contraception, and are similar to the recurrent jaundice of pregnancy, i.e. benign and reversible. The incidence with lower dose oral contraception is unknown, but it must be a rare occurrence.

The only absolute hepatic contraindication to oral contraceptive use is acute or chronic cholestatic liver disease. Cirrhosis and previous hepatitis are not aggravated. Once recovered from the acute phase of liver disease, a woman can use oral contraception.

The Gallbladder

The incidence of gallstones in early reports from Britain indicated an increased incidence after the first 2 years of use, with a return to the level of the control group after 4 years. The latest British data, however, have indicated that this apparent increase was due to an acceleration of gallbladder disease in women already susceptible.[69] In other words, the overall risk of gallbladder disease is not increased, but in the first years of use, disease is activated or accelerated in women who are vulnerable because of asymptomatic disease or a tendency toward gallbladder disease. The mechanism appears to be induced alterations in the composition of gallbladder bile, specifically a rise in cholesterol saturation that is presumably an estrogen effect.[70] One anticipates a lesser effect in the forthcoming reports describing the effects of low dose pills. Keep in mind that while studies have found a statistically significant increase in the relative risk of gallbladder disease, because the actual incidence of this problem is low, the effect is of minimal clinical importance.

Other Metabolic Effects

Nausea, breast discomfort, and weight gain continue to be disturbing effects, but their incidence is significantly less with low dose oral contraception. Fortunately, these effects are most intense in the first few months of use, and in most cases, gradually disappear. Weight gain usually responds to dietary restriction, but for some patients, the weight gain is an anabolic response to the sex steroids, and discontinuation of oral contraception is the only way that weight loss can be achieved. This must be rare with low dose oral contraception because the data in published studies fail to indicate a difference between users and nonusers.

Chloasma, a patchy increase in facial pigment, was, at one time, found to occur in approximately 5% of oral contraceptive users. It is now a rare problem due to the decrease in estrogen dose. Unfortunately, once chloasma appears, it fades only gradually following discontinuation of the pill, and may never disappear completely. Skin blanching medications may be useful.

Hematologic effects include an increased sedimentation rate due to increased levels of fibrinogen, increased total iron binding capacity due to the increase in globulins, and a decrease in prothrombin time. The continuous use of oral contraceptives may prevent the appearance of symptoms in porphyria precipitated by menses. Changes in vitamin metabolism have been noted: a small nonharmful increase in Vitamin A, decreases in blood levels of pyridoxine (B_6) and the other B vitamins, folic acid, and ascorbic acid. Despite these changes, routine vitamin supplements have not been shown to be of benefit for women eating adequate, normal diets.

In well-controlled studies, no increases in eye abnormalities have been detected in oral contraceptive users (contrary to early anecdotal reports). Rarely, mental depression is associated with oral contraceptives. In studies with higher dose oral contraceptives, the effect was due to estrogen interference with the synthesis of tryptophan which could be reversed with pyridoxine treatment. It seems wiser, however, to discontinue oral contraception if depression is encountered. Though infrequent, a reduction in libido is occasionally a problem, and may be a cause for seeking an alternative method of contraception.

Because estrogen is known to stimulate prolactin secretion and to cause hypertrophy of the pituitary lactotrophs, it was appropriate to be concerned over a possible relationship between oral contraception and prolactin-secreting pituitary adenomas. Several case-control studies have uniformly concluded that no such relationship exists. There is insufficient information regarding the effect of oral contraceptives on existing prolactinomas, although at least one study demonstrated that previous use of oral contraceptives had no effect on the size of prolactinomas.[71] We have routinely prescribed oral contraception to patients with pituitary microadenomas and have never observed evidence of tumor growth.

The Risk of Cancer

Endometrial Cancer

The use of oral contraception protects against endometrial cancer. Use for at least 12 months reduces the risk of developing endometrial cancer by 50%, with the greatest protective effect gained by use greater than 3 years.[72] This protection persists for 15 or more years after discontinuation (the actual length of duration of protection is unknown), and is greatest in women at highest risk: nulliparous and low parity women. This protection is equally protective for all 3 major histologic subtypes of endometrial cancer: adenocarcinoma, adenoacanthoma, and adenosquamous cancers. Finally, protection is seen with all monophasic formulations of oral contraceptives, including pills with less than 50 μg of estrogen. There are no data as yet with multiphasic preparations, but since the multiphasic pills are still dominated by their progestational component, there is every reason to believe that they will be protective.

Ovarian Cancer

Protection against ovarian cancer, the most lethal of female reproductive tract cancers, is one of the most important benefits of oral contraception. Because this cancer is detected late and prognosis is poor, the impact of this protection is very significant. The risk of developing epithelial ovarian cancer in users of oral contraception is reduced by 40% compared to that of nonusers.[73] This protective effect increases with duration of use (taking 5–10 years to become apparent) and continues for at least 10–15 years after stopping the medication. This protection is seen in women who use oral contraception for as little as 3 to 6 months, reaches an 80% reduction in risk with more than 10 years of use, and it is a benefit associated with all monophasic formulations. Again, the multiphasic pills have not been in use long enough to yield any data on this issue, but because ovulation is effectively inhibited by the multiphasics, protection against ovarian cancer should be exerted.

In the 1980s, approximately 2000 cases of endometrial cancer and 1700 cases of ovarian cancer were averted annually in the United States by past and current users of oral contraception.

Cancer of the Cervix

Studies have indicated that the risk for dysplasia and carcinoma-in-situ of the uterine cervix increases with the use of oral contraception for more than one year.[74] Invasive cervical cancer may be increased after 5 years of use, reaching a two-fold increase after 10 years. It is well recognized, however, that the number of partners a woman has had and age at first coitus are the most important risk factors for cervical neoplasia. Other confounding factors include exposure to human papillomavirus, the use of barrier contraception (protective), and smoking. These are difficult factors to control, and therefore, the conclusions regarding cervical cancer are not definitive. An excellent study from the Centers for Disease Control concluded there is no increased risk of invasive cervical cancer in uses of oral contraception, and an apparent increased risk of carcinoma-in-situ is due to enhanced detection of disease (because oral contraceptive users have more frequent Pap smears).[75] On the other hand, an excellent case-control study of patients in Panama, Costa Rica, Colombia, and Mexico concluded that there is a minimal risk for invasive squamous cell carcinoma (RR = 1.1), but there is a significantly increased risk for invasive adenocarcinoma (RR = 2.4).[76]

This concern obviously is an important reason for annual Pap smear surveillance. Fortunately, steroid contraception does not mask abnormal cervical changes, and the necessity for prescription renewals offers the opportunity for improved screening for cervical disease. We believe it is reasonable to perform Pap smears every 6 months in women using oral contraception for 5 or more years who are also at higher risk because of their sexual behavior (multiple partners, history of sexually transmitted diseases).

Neoplasia of the Liver

Liver Adenomas. Hepatocellular adenomas can be produced by steroids of both the estrogen and androgen families. Actually, there are two different lesions, peliosis and adenomas. Peliosis is characterized by dilated vascular spaces without endothelial lining, and may occur in the absence of adenomatous changes. The adenomas are not malignant; their significance lies in the potential for hemorrhage. The most common presentation is acute right upper quadrant or epigastric pain. The tumors may be asymptomatic, or they may present suddenly with hematoperitoneum. There is some evidence that the tumors regress when oral contraception is stopped. Epidemiologic data have not supported the contention that mestranol increased the risk more than ethinyl estradiol.

The risk appears to be related to duration of oral contraceptive use and to the steroid dose in the pills. This is reinforced by the rarity of the condition ever since low dose oral contraception became available. The ongoing prospective studies have accumulated many woman-years of use and have not identified a single case of such a tumor. In our view it isn't even worth mentioning during the informed consent (choice) process.

No reliable screening test or procedure is currently available. Routine liver function tests are normal. CT scanning may be the best means of diagnosis; angiography and ultrasonography are not reliable. Palpation of the liver should be part of the periodic evaluation in oral contraceptive users. If an enlarged liver is found, oral contraception should be stopped, and regression should be evaluated and followed by CT scan.

Liver Cancer. Oral contraception has been linked to the development of hepatocellular carcinoma.[77,78] However, the very small number of cases, and thus the limited statistical power, requires great caution in interpretation. The largest study on this question, the WHO Collaborative Study of Neoplasia and Steroid Contraceptives, found no association between oral contraception and liver cancer.[79] In the United States, the death rates from liver cancer have not changed over the last 3 decades despite introduction and widespread use of oral contraception.

Breast Cancer

One of every 9 American women will develop breast cancer during her lifetime. The incidence has been increasing over the past 2 decades and mortality rates have remained disappointingly constant. The breast is the leading site of cancer in women (28% of all cancers), but smoking has now made lung cancer the leading cause of death from cancer in women.

Because of its prevalence and its long latent phase, it is not surprising that concern over the relationship between oral contraception and breast cancer continues to be an issue in the minds of both patients and clinicians. Unfortunately, the issue is not resolved and probably will not be until another decade passes, allowing data to emerge from the modern era of lower dose oral contraception.

Worth emphasizing is the protective effect of higher dose oral contraception on benign breast disease, an effect which becomes apparent after 2 years of use.[80] After 2 years there is a progressive reduction (about 40%) in the incidence of fibrocystic disease of the breast. Women who used oral contraception were one-fourth as likely to develop benign breast disease as nonusers, but this protection was limited to current and recent users. It is still unkown whether this same protection is provided by the lower dose products.

The RCGP[11], OFPA[81,82], and Walnut Creek[16] cohort studies (and more recently, the Nurses' Health Study[83]) indicated no significant differences in breast cancer rates between users and nonusers. However, patients were enrolled in these studies at a time when oral contraception was used primarily by married couples spacing out their children. By the 1980s, oral contraception was primarily being used by women early in life, for longer durations, and to delay an initial pregnancy (remember, a full-term pregnancy early in life protects against breast cancer).

Over the last decade, case-control studies have focused on the use of oral contraception early in life, for long duration, and to delay a first, full-term pregnancy. Because the cohort of women who have used oral contraception in this fashion is just now beginning to reach the ages of postmenopausal breast cancer, the studies had to examine the risk of breast cancer diagnosed before age 45 (only 13% of all breast cancer).

Some studies have indicated an overall increased relative risk of early, premenopausal breast cancer[84–89], while others indicated no increase in overall risk.[90–99] However, each of these studies suffers from the problems encountered by case-control studies of a difficult subject: differences in controls, small numbers of cases, a small percentage of women who used oral contraception for long durations.

Examining use before a first full-term pregnancy again does not yield consistent results. Some studies indicate an increased risk for breast cancer[85,87,95,100], but most do not.[84,88,89,94,96,97,98,101] Here too, there are the same concerns. For example, in the OFPA study, the relative risk for use before a first full-term pregnancy was 2.59, however, only 2% of their patients used oral contraception before a first full-term pregnancy.[95] For use before age 25, the majority of studies, but not all, indicated no increased risk of breast cancer. The most impressive finding indicates a link in most studies[85,87,88,95,96,100] but not all[97,98], of early breast cancer before age 40 in women who used oral contraception for long durations of time. On the other hand, we have situations such as a positive report in which only 14 women had breast cancer and there were only 15 woman-years of use before age 20.[95]

The Centers for Disease Control study is the largest case-control study on the subject.[102–104] No overall increased risk of breast cancer was found in women using oral contraceptives before the age of 20 with a duration of use greater than 4 years, or before the age of 25 with a duration of use greater than 6 years, or with greater than 4 years use before a first pregnancy. In addition, no overall increased risk of breast cancer was found among any subgroups of users including women with benign breast disease or a family history of breast cancer.

In further analysis of the CDC study, there was no increased risk associated with any specific type of oral contraceptive, progestin only pills, or the use of 2 or more types. In addition, there was no increased risk associated with any specific progestin or estrogen component, and most importantly, it was demonstrated that long-term use (15 or more years) was not associated with an increased risk of breast cancer. The reliability of the CDC study is reinforced by the fact that the data confirmed the previously identified risk factors, such as nulliparity, late age at first birth, history of benign breast disease, and a family history of breast cancer. Thus far, the CDC study has found no evidence for a latent effect (increased risk many years later) on breast cancer risk through age 54.[105]

In view of the confusing and contradictory findings among the many case-control studies, the CDC reexamined their data to determine whether oral contraceptive use had different effects on the risk of breast cancer diagnosed at different ages.[106] The data indicated that oral contraceptive use increased slightly the risk of breast cancer diagnosed under the age of 35, had no effect on women diagnosed from age 35 to 44, and in women diagnosed from age 45 to 54, oral contraceptive use appeared to decrease the risk of breast cancer. However, these estimates were of borderline statistical significance. Nevertheless, the protection that oral contraceptive use appears to provide to older women is a more convincing argument because it was supported by several dose-response relationships (age with first use and time since first and last use). The elevated risk among the women with early breast cancer is a more tenuous conclusion, not strengthened by supporting dose-response patterns.

The crucial question is: as studies gain more statistical power, will they confirm a slightly increased risk for premenopausal breast cancer or will the present suggestion of an increased risk disappear? For example, an early report from New Zealand indicated an increased relative risk for premenopausal breast cancer, and as the study continues, this relative risk is moving closer and closer to 1.0.[107] This excellent New Zealand study reports no increase in risk of breast cancer associated with long duration of use, use before a first full term pregnancy, or use at a young age.

59

Further comfort can be derived from the United States national cancer surveillance data.[108] The increase in breast cancer in American women is in older women, those who did not have the opportunity to use oral contraception. In women under 56 years of age, there has been no change in the age-specific breast cancer rates from 1950 to 1985.

Since oral contraceptive use decreases benign breast disease and benign breast disease increases a woman's risk of breast cancer, why doesn't oral contraception decrease the risk of breast cancer? It has been argued that the impact of oral contraception on benign breast disease must be limited to the type of tissue change that is not linked to breast cancer risk. It is also possible that oral contraception either accelerates the development of breast cancer that would have been diagnosed later, or leads to earlier diagnosis through greater involvement with a health care system, or perhaps both of these.

Conclusion. For some time to come, probably a decade or more, clinical advice will have to be based on the current conflicting findings. With considerable confidence, we believe that long-term use of oral contraception during the reproductive years is NOT associated with a significant increase in the risk of breast cancer after age 45. There is the possibility that a subgroup of young women who use contraception early and for a long time (greater than 4 years) has a slightly increased risk of breast cancer before the age of 45, a relative risk of less than 1.5. It is not cost effective to promote mammographic surveillance of this group of patients, but it should not be denied to any woman of this group who makes the request. There is also the possibility that previous users of oral contraception are provided some protection against postmenopausal breast cancer. Keep in mind that these conclusions depend upon data derived from use of higher dose oral contraception. It is important to be aware that there has been consistent failure to demonstrate an increased risk with oral contraceptive use in women with positive family histories of breast cancer or in women with proven benign breast disease.[103,107,109]

Adding up the benefits of oral contraception, the possible slight increase in risk of breast cancer is far outweighed by positive effects on our public health. But the impact on public health is of little concern during the private clinician-patient interchange in the office. Here personal risk receives highest priority; fear of cancer is a motivating force, and compliance with effective contraception requires accurate information.

The clinician should not fail to take every opportunity to direct attention to all factors that affect breast cancer. Breastfeeding and control of alcohol intake are good examples, and are also components of preventive health care. Especially important is this added motivation to encourage breastfeeding. The protective effect of breast feeding is greatest for premenopausal breast cancer, the cancer of concern to younger women using oral contraception.

Patients deserve to know the facts and need help in dealing with the state of the art and the uncertainty. But there is no doubt that patients, especially young patients, are influenced in their choice by their clinician's advice and attitude. We are concerned over the findings of the breast cancer reports, but the definitive answer awaits future studies. We believe the safety and benefits of low dose oral contraception currently outweigh the potential risks.

Other Cancers

The Walnut Creek study suggested that melanoma was linked to oral contraception, however, the major risk factor for melanoma is exposure to sunlight. More recent and accurate evaluation utilizing both of the RCGP and OFPA prospective cohorts and accounting for exposure to sunlight, has not indicated a significant difference in the risk of melanoma comparing users to nonusers.[110,111] There is no evidence linking oral contraceptive use to kidney cancer, colon cancer, gallbladder cancer, or pituitary tumors.[112]

Endocrine Effects

Adrenal Gland

For some time it has been known that estrogen increases the cortisol-binding globulin, transcortin. It had been thought that the increase in plasma cortisol while on oral contraception was due to increased binding by this globulin and not an increase in free active cortisol. Now it is apparent that free and active cortisol levels are also elevated. Estrogen decreases the ability of the liver to metabolize cortisol, and in addition, progesterone and related compounds can displace cortisol from transcortin, and thus contribute to the elevation of unbound cortisol. The effects of these elevated levels over prolonged periods of time are unknown. To put this into perspective, the increase is not as great as that which occurs in pregnancy, and, in fact, it is within the normal range for nonpregnant women.

The adrenal gland responds to adrenocorticotropic hormone (ACTH) normally in women on oral contraceptives, therefore there is no suppression of the adrenal gland itself. Initial studies showed that the response to metyrapone (11β hydroxylase blocker) was abnormal, suggesting that the pituitary was suppressed. However estrogen accelerates the conjugation of metyrapone by the liver, and therefore the drug has less effect, thus explaining the subnormal responses initially reported. The pituitary-adrenal reaction to stress is normal in women on oral contraceptive pills.

Thyroid

As with transcortin, estrogen increases thyroxine-binding globulin, Prior to the introduction of new methods for measuring free thyroxine levels, evaluation of thyroid function was a problem. Measurement of TSH (thyroid stimulating hormone) and the free thyroxine level in a woman on oral contraception now provides an accurate assessment of a patient's thyroid state. Oral contraception affects the total thyroxine level in the blood as well as the amount of binding globulin, but the free thyroxine level is unchanged.

Oral Contraception and Reproduction

The impact of oral contraceptives on the reproductive system is less than initially thought. Early studies which indicated adverse effects have not stood the test of time and the scrutiny of multiple, careful studies. There are two major areas which deserve review: (1). Inadvertent use of oral contraceptives during the cycle of conception and during early pregnancy, and (2). Reproduction after discontinuing oral contraception.

Inadvertent Use During the Cycle of Conception and During Early Pregnancy

One of the reasons, if not the major reason, why a lack of withdrawal bleeding while using oral contraceptives is such a problem is the anxiety produced in both patient and clinician. The patient is anxious because of the uncertainty regarding pregnancy, and the clinician is anxious because of the concerns stemming from the retrospective studies which indicated an increased risk of congenital malformations among the offspring of women who were pregnant and using oral contraception.

Organogenesis does not occur in the first 2 embryonic weeks (first 4 weeks since last menstrual period), however teratogenic effects are possible between the third and eighth embryonic weeks (5 to 10 weeks since LMP).

Initial positive reports linking the use of contraceptive steroids to congenital malformations have not been substantiated. Many suspect a strong component of recall bias in the few positive studies due to a tendency of patients with malformed infants to recall details better than those with normal children. Other confounding problems have included a failure to consider the reasons for the administration of hormones (e.g. bleeding in an already abnormal pregnancy), and a failure to delineate the exact timing of the treatment (e.g. treatment was sometimes confined to a period of time during which the heart could not have been affected).

An association with cardiac anomalies was first claimed in the 1970s.[113,114] This link received considerable support with a report from the U.S. Collaborative Perinatal Project, subsequently analysis of these data uncovered several methodologic shortcomings.[115] Simpson, in a very thorough and critical review in 1990, concluded that there is no reliable evidence implicating sex steroids as cardiac teratogens.[116] In fact, in his review, Simpson found no relationship between oral contraception and the following problems: hypospadias, limb reduction anomalies, neural tube defects, and mutagenic effects which would be responsible for chromosomally abnormal fetuses. Even virilization is not a practical consideration because the doses required (e.g. 20–40 mg norethindrone per day) are in excess of anything currently used. These conclusions reflect use of combined oral contraceptives as well as progestins alone.

In the past there was a concern regarding the VACTERL complex. VACTERL refers to a complex of vertebral, anal, cardiac, tracheoesophageal, renal, and limb anomalies. While case-control studies indicated a relationship with oral contraception, prospective studies have failed to observe any connection between sex steroids and the VACTERL complex.[117,118] A meta-analysis of 26 prospective studies of the risk of birth defects with oral contraceptive ingestion during pregnancy concluded that there was no increase in risk for major malformations, congenital heart defects, or limb reduction defects.[119]

Women who become pregnant while taking oral contraceptives or women who inadvertently take birth control pills early in pregnancy should be advised that the risk of a significant congenital anomaly is no greater than the general rate of 2–3%. This recommendation can be extended to those pregnant woman who have been exposed to a progestational agent such as medroxyprogesterone acetate or 17-hydroxyprogesterone caproate.[120,121]

Reproduction after Discontinuing Oral Contraception

Fertility. The early reports from the English prospective studies indicated that former users of oral contraception had a delay in achieving pregnancy. In the OFPA study, former use had an effect on fertility for up to 42 months in nulligravida women and for up to 30 months in multigravida women.[122] Presumably the delay is due to lingering suppression of the hypothalamic-pituitary reproductive system.

A later analysis of the Oxford data indicated that the delay is concentrated in women age 30–34 who have never given birth.[123] At 48 months 82% of these women had given birth compared to 89% of users of other contraceptive methods. No effect was observed in women younger than 30 or in women who had previously given birth. Childless women age 25–29 experienced some delay in return to fertility, but by 48 months, 91% had given birth compared to 92% in users of other methods. It should be noted that after 72 months the proportions of women who remained undelivered were the same in both groups of women.

This delay has been observed in the United States as well. In the Boston area, the interval from cessation of contraception to conception was 13 months or greater for 24.8% of prior oral contraceptive users compared to 10.6% for former users of all other methods (12.4% for IUD users, 8.5% for diaphragm uses, and 11.9% for other methods).[124] Oral contraceptive users had a lower monthly percentage of conceptions for the first 3 months, and somewhat lower percentage from 4 to 10 months. It took 24 months for 90% of previous oral contraceptive users to become pregnant, 14 months for IUD users, and 10 months for diaphragm users. Similar findings in Connecticut indicate that this delay lasts at least a year, and the effect is greater with higher dose preparations.[125] Despite this delay, there is no evidence that infertility is increased by the use of oral contraception.

64

Spontaneous Abortion. There is no increase in the incidence of spontaneous abortion in pregnancies after the cessation of oral contraception.[126] Indeed, The rate of spontaneous abortion and stillbirths is slightly less in former pill users, about 1% less for spontaneous abortions and 0.3% less for stillbirths.

Pregnancy Outcome. There is no evidence that oral contraceptives cause changes in individual germ cells that would yield an abnormal child at a later time.[116] There is no increase in the number of abnormal children born to former oral contraceptive users, and there is no change in the sex ratio (a sign of sex-linked recessive mutations).[127] These observations are not altered when analyzed for duration of use. Initial observations that women who had previously used oral contraception had an increase in chromosomally abnormal fetuses have not been confirmed. Furthermore, as noted above, there is no increase in the abortion rate after discontinuation, something one would expect if oral contraceptives induce chromosomal abnormalities since these are the principal cause of spontaneous abortion.

In a 3 year follow-up of children whose mothers used oral contraceptives prior to conception, no differences could be detected in weight, anemia, intelligence, or development.[128] Former oral contraceptive users have no increased risks for the following: perinatal morbidity or mortality, prematurity, and low birth weight.[129,130] Dizygous twinning has been observed to be nearly two-fold (1.6% vs 1.0%) increased in women who conceive soon after cessation of oral contraception.[126] This effect was greater with greater duration of use.

The only reason (and it is a good one) to recommend that women defer attempts to conceive for a month or two after stopping oral contraception is to improve the accuracy of gestational dating by allowing accurate identification of the last menstrual period.

Breastfeeding. Oral contraception has been demonstrated to diminish the quantity and quality of lactation in postpartum women. Also of concern is the potential hazard of transfer of contraceptive steroids to the infant (a significant amount of the progestational component is transferred into breast milk)[131], however no adverse effects have thus far been identified. Women who use oral contraception have a lower incidence of breastfeeding after the 6th postpartum month, regardless of whether oral contraception is started at the first, second, or third postpartum month.[132–134]

In adequately nourished women, no impairment of infant growth can be detected; presumably compensation is achieved either through supplementary feedings or increased suckling.[135] In an 8 year follow-up study of children breastfed by mothers using oral contraceptives, no effect could be detected on diseases, intelligence, or psychological behavior.[136] This study also found that mothers on birth control pills lactated a significantly shorter period of time than controls, a mean of 3.7 months vs 4.6 months in controls.

Because the above considerations indicate that oral contraception shortens the duration of breastfeeding, it is worthwhile to consider the contraceptive effectiveness of lactation. In Scotland, no ovulation could be detected in women during exclusive breastfeeding.[137] However, in Chile, 14% of women ovulated during full breastfeeding, although full nursing provided effective contraception up to 3 months postpartum.[138,139] It has been argued that the threshold for suppression of ovulation is at least 5 feedings for a total of at least 65 minutes per day of suckling duration.[140] However in the studies from Chile, the frequency of nursing was the same in breastfeeders who ovulated and those who did not.

In Mexico, a study of 29 breastfeeding mothers and 10 nonbreastfeeders observed that in the absence of bleeding and supplementary feedings, 100% of the breastfeeders remained anovulatory for 3 months postpartum, and 96% up to 6 months.[141] The median time from delivery to first ovulation was 259 days for breastfeeders compared to 119 days for nonbreastfeeders. However, by the third postpartum month, 18% of the breastfeeders had ovulated. Only amenorrheic women who exclusively breastfeed at regular intervals, including nighttime, during the first 6 months have the contraceptive protection equivalent to that provided by oral contraception; with menstruation or after 6 months, the risk of ovulation increases.[142] Supplemental feeding increases the risk of ovulation (and pregnancy) even in amenorrheic women.[143] Total protection against pregnancy is achieved by the exclusively breastfeeding woman for a duration of only 10 weeks.

It is apparent that while lactation provides a contraceptive effect, it is variable and not reliable for every woman. Furthermore, because frequent suckling is required to maintain full milk production, women who use oral contraception and also breastfeed less frequently (e.g. because they work outside their home) have two reasons for decreased milk volume. This combination can make it especially difficult to continue nursing.

Because of the concerns regarding the impact of oral contraceptives on breastfeeding, a useful alternative is to combine the contraceptive effect of lactation with the progestin-only minipill.(see Chapters 3 and 8) This low dose of progestin has no negative impact on breast milk, and some studies document an increase in milk quantity and nutritional quality. Highly effective (near total) protection can be achieved with the combination of lactation and the minipill.

Other Considerations

Prolactin-Secreting Adenomas.   Because estrogen is known to stimulate prolactin secretion and to cause hypertrophy of the pituitary lactotrophs, it is appropriate to be concerned over a possible relationship between oral contraception and prolactin-secreting adenomas. Several case-control studies have uniformly concluded that no such relationship exists.[144,145] Data from both the RCGP and the OFPA studies indicated no increase in the incidence of pituitary adenomas.[112,146] There is insufficient information regarding the effect of oral contraceptives on existing prolactinomas, although one study demonstrated that previous use of oral contraceptives had no effect on the size of prolactinomas.[71] *We have routinely prescribed oral contraception to patients with pituitary microadenomas and have never observed evidence of tumor growth.*

Postpill Amenorrhea.   The approximate incidence of "postpill amenorrhea" is 0.7–0.8%, which is equal to the incidence of spontaneous secondary amenorrhea[130,147,148], and there is no evidence to support the idea that oral contraception causes secondary amenorrhea. If a cause and effect relationship exists between oral contraception and subsequent amenorrhea, one would expect the incidence of infertility to be increased after a given population discontinues use of oral contraception. In those women who discontinue oral contraception in order to get pregnant, 50% conceive by 3 months, and after 2 years, a maximum of 15% of nulliparous women and 7% of parous women fail to conceive[130], figures comparable to those quoted for the prevalence of spontaneous infertility. Attempts to document a cause and effect relationship between oral contraceptive use and secondary amenorrhea have failed.[149] While patients with this problem come more quickly to our attention because of previous oral contraceptive use and follow-up, there is no cause and effect relationship. Women who have not resumed menstrual function within 12 months should be evaluated as any other patient with secondary amenorrhea.

Use During Puberty. An important related question is: should oral contraception be advised for a young woman with irregular menses and oligoovulation or anovulation? The fear of subsequent infertility should not be a deterrent to providing appropriate contraception. Women who have irregular menstrual periods are more likely to develop secondary amenorrhea whether they use oral contraception or not. The possibility of subsequent secondary amenorrhea is less of a risk and a less urgent problem for a young woman than leaving her unprotected. The need for contraception takes precedence.

There is no evidence that the use of oral contraceptives in the pubertal, sexually active girl impairs growth and development of the reproductive system. Again, the most important concern is and should be the prevention of an unwanted pregnancy. For most teenagers oral contraception, dispensed in the 28-day package for better compliance, is the contraceptive method of choice.

The Postpartum Visit. The individual woman is in need of contraception early in the postpartum period. In a careful study of 22 postpartum, nonbreastfeeding women, the mean time from delivery to the first menses was 45 ± 10.1 days, and no woman ovulated before 25 days after delivery.[150] A high proportion of the first cycles (81.8%) and the subsequent cycles (37%) were not normal, however this is certainly not predictable in individual women. Others have documented a mean delay of 7 weeks before resumption of ovulation, but half of the women studied ovulated before the 6th week, the time of the traditional postpartum visit. *The obstetrical tradition of scheduling the postpartum visit at 6 weeks should be changed. A 3-week visit would be more effective for avoiding postpartum surprises.*

After the termination of a pregnancy of less than 12 weeks, oral contraception can be started immediately. After a pregnancy of 12 or more weeks, oral contraception has traditionally been started 2 weeks after delivery to avoid an increased risk of thrombosis during the initial postpartum period. This practice has been based on a theoretical concern which is probably no longer an issue with low dose oral contraception. We believe that oral contraception can be started immediately after a second trimester abortion or premature delivery.

Infections and Oral Contraception

Bacterial STDs

Sexually transmitted diseases (STDs) are one of the most common public health problems in the United States. Approximately 1 million cases of pelvic inflammatory disease (PID) occur annually in the United States.[151] This upper genital tract infection is usually a consequence of STDs. The best estimate of subsequent tubal infertility is derived from an excellent Swedish report; approximately 12% after one episode of PID, 23% after 2 episodes, and 54% after 3 episodes.[152] Because pelvic infection is the single greatest threat to the reproductive future of a young woman, the now recognized protection offered by oral contraception against pelvic inflammatory disease is highly important.[153-156] The risk of hospitalization for PID is reduced by approximately 50%–60%, but at least 12 months of use are necessary, and the protection is limited to current users.[154,157] Furthermore, if a patient does get a pelvic infection, the severity of the salpingitis found at laparoscopy is decreased.[158] The mechanism of this protection remains unknown. Speculation includes thickening of the cervical mucus to prevent movement of pathogens and bacteria-laden sperm into the uterus and tubes, and decreased menstrual bleeding reducing movement of pathogens into the tubes as well as a reduction in "culture medium."

Recently the argument has been made that this protection is limited to gonococcal disease, and chlamydial infections may even be enhanced. Fifteen of 17 published studies by 1985 reported a positive association of oral contraceptives with lower genital tract chlamydial cervicitis.[159] Because lower genital tract infections caused by chlamydia are on the rise (now the most prevalent bacterial STD in the U.S.) and the rate of hospitalization for PID is also increased, it is worthwhile for both patients and clinicians to be alert for symptoms of cervicitis or salpingitis in women on oral contraception who are at high risk of sexually transmitted disease (multiple sexual partners, a history of STD, or cervical discharge).

Despite this potential relationship between oral contraception and chlamydial infections, it should be emphasized that there is no evidence for an impact of oral contraceptives increasing the incidence of tubal infertility.[160] In fact, a case-control study indicates that oral contraceptive users with chlamydia infection are protected against symptomatic PID.[161] Thus, the influence of oral contraception on the upper reproductive tract may be different than on the lower tract. These observations on fertility are derived mostly, if not totally, from women using oral contraceptives containing 50 µg of estrogen. The continued progestin dominance of the lower dose formulations, however, should produce the same protective impact, and evidence is appearing that this is so.[157]

Viral STDs

The viral STDs include human immunodeficiency virus (HIV), human papillomavirus (HPV), herpes simplex virus (HSV), and hepatitis B (HBV). At the present time, no known associations exist between oral contraception and the viral STDs.[162] Of course, significant prevention includes barrier methods of contraception (see Chapter 6). Thus far, most studies have found no association beween oral contraceptive use and HIV seropositivity. *For women not in a stable, monogamous relationship, a dual approach is recommended, combining the contraceptive efficacy and protection against PID offered by oral contraception with the use of a barrier method (and spermicide) for prevention of viral STDs.*

Other Infections

In the British prospective studies, urinary tract infections were increased in users of oral contraception by 20%, and a correlation was noted with estrogen dose. An increased incidence of cervicitis was also reported, an effect related to the progestin dose. The incidence of cervicitis increased with the length of time the pill was used, from no higher after 6 months to 3 times higher by the 6th year of use. A significant increase in a variety of viral diseases, e.g. chickenpox, was observed, suggesting steroid effects on the immune system. The prevalence of these effects with low dose oral contraception is yet unknown.

Oral contraception is not linked to bacterial vaginosis, but appears to protect against infections with *Trichomonas*.[163] Evidence is lacking to convincingly implicate oral contraception with vaginal infections with *Candida* species[163], however, clinical experience is sometimes impressive when recurrence and cure repeatedly follow use and discontinuation of oral contraception.

Patient Management

Absolute Contraindications to the Use of Oral Contraception

1. Thrombophlebitis, thromboembolic disorders, cerebral vascular disease, coronary occlusion, or a past history of these conditions, or conditions predisposing to these problems.
2. Markedly impaired liver function. Steroid hormones are contraindicated in patients with hepatitis until liver function tests return to normal.
3. Known or suspected breast cancer.
4. Undiagnosed abnormal vaginal bleeding.
5. Known or suspected pregnancy.
6. Smokers over the age of 35.

Relative Contraindications Requiring Clinical Judgment and Informed Consent

1. Migraine headaches. In retrospective studies of high dose pills, migraine headaches have been associated with an increased risk of stroke, however some women report an improvement in their headaches.
2. Hypertension. A woman under 35 who is otherwise healthy and whose blood pressure is controlled by medication can elect to use oral contraception.
3. Uterine leiomyoma. This is no longer a contraindication with the low dose formulations. There is evidence that the risk of leiomyomas is decreased by 31% in women who used higher dose oral contraception for 10 years.[164]
4. Gestational diabetes. Low dose formulations do not produce a diabetic glucose tolerance response in women with previous gestational diabetes, and there is no evidence that oral contraception increases the incidence of overt diabetes mellitus. We believe that women with previous gestational diabetes can use oral contraception with annual assessment of the fasting glucose level.
5. Elective surgery. The recommendation that oral contraception should be discontinued 4 weeks before elective surgery to avoid an increased risk of postoperative thrombosis is based upon data derived from high dose pills. If possible, it is safer to follow this recommendation, but it is probably less critical with low dose oral contraceptives. It is more prudent to maintain contra-

ception right up to the performance of a sterilization procedure, and this short, outpatient operation probably carries very minimal risk.

6. Epilepsy. Oral contraceptives do not exacerbate epilepsy, and in some women, improvement in seizure control has occurred.[165] Antiepileptic drugs, however, may decrease the effectiveness of oral contraception.
7. Obstructive jaundice in pregnancy. Not all patients with this history will develop jaundice on oral contraception, especially with the low dose formulations.
8. Sickle cell disease or sickle C disease. Patients with sickle cell trait can use oral contraception. The risk of thrombosis in women with sickle cell disease or sickle C diseases is theoretical (and medical-legal). We believe effective protection against pregnancy in these patients warrants the use of low dose oral contraception.
9. Diabetes mellitus. Effective prevention of pregnancy outweighs the small risk in diabetic women who are under age 35 and otherwise healthy.
10. Gallbladder disease.

Clinical Decisions

Surveillance. Previously patients have been monitored every 6 months while on oral contraception. In view of the increased safety of low dose preparations for healthy young women with no risk factors, patients need be seen only every 12 months for exclusion of problems by history, measurement of the blood pressure, urinalysis, breast examination, palpation of the liver, and pelvic examination with Pap smear. Women with risk factors should be seen every 6 months by appropriately trained personnel for screening of problems by history and blood pressure measurement. Breast and pelvic examinations are necessary only yearly. It is worth emphasizing that better compliance is achieved by reassessing new users within 3 months. It is at this time that subtle fears and unvoiced concerns need to be confronted and resolved.

Oral contraception is safer than we thought it was, and the low dose preparations are extremely safe. Health care providers should make a significant effort to get this message to our patients (and our colleagues). We must make sure our patients receive adequate counseling, either from ourselves or our professional staff. The major reason why patients discontinue oral contraception is fear of side effects.[166] Let's take time to put the risks into proper perspective, and to emphasize the benefits as well as the risks.

Laboratory surveillance should be used only when indicated. Routine biochemical measurements fail to yield sufficient information to warrant the expense. Assessing the cholesterol-lipoprotein profile and carbohydrate metabolism should follow the same guidelines applied to all patients, users and nonusers of contraception. The following is a useful guide as to who should be monitored with blood screening tests for glucose, lipids, and lipoproteins:

> Young women, at least once.
> Women 35 years or older.
> Women with a strong family history of heart disease, diabetes mellitus, or hypertension.
> Women with gestational diabetes melllitus.
> Women with xanthomatosis.
> Obese women.
> Diabetic women.

Choice of Pill. The therapeutic principle remains: utilize the formulations which give effective contraception and the greatest margin of safety. The multiphasic preparations do have a reduced progestin dosage compared to some of the existing monophasic products, however, based on currently available information there is little difference between the low dose monophasics and the multiphasics. It remains to be seen whether formulations with the new progestins will provide protection against cardiovascular disease, nevertheless the new progestin combinations offer minimal metabolic impact (although it is by no means certain yet that this impact is better than the available low dose formulations). The one exception is monophasic preparations containing relatively high doses of levonorgestrel, 150–250 μg; these should be avoided in favor of low dose formulations.

You and your patients are urged to choose a low dose preparation containing less than 50 μg of estrogen, combined with low doses of new or old progestins, avoiding the high doses of levonorgestrel. Current data support the view that there is greater safety with preparations containing less than 50 μg of estrogen. The arguments in this chapter indicate that all patients should begin oral contraception with low dose products, and that patients on higher dose oral contraception should be changed to the low dose preparations.

Stepping down to a lower dose can be accomplished immediately with no adverse reactions such as increased bleeding or failure of contraception.

The pharmacologic effects in animals of various formulations have been used as a basis for therapeutic recommendations in selecting the optimal oral contraceptive pill. *These recommendations (tailor-making the pill to the patient) have not been supported by appropriately controlled clinical trials. All too often this leads to the prescribing of a pill of excessive dosage with its attendant increased risk of serious side effects.* It is worth repeating our earlier comments on potency. Oral contraceptive potency (specifically progestin potency) is no longer a consideration when it comes to prescribing birth control pills. The potency of the various progestins has been accounted for by appropriate adjustments of dose. Clinical advice based on potency is an artificial exercise which has not stood the test of time. The biologic effect of the various progestational components in current low dose oral contraceptives is approximately the same. Our progress in lowering the doses of the steroids contained in oral contraceptives has yielded products with little serious differences.

Pill Taking. Effective contraception is present during the first cycle of pill use, provided the pills are started no later than the 5th day of the cycle, and no pills are missed. Thus, starting oral contraception on the first day of menses assures immediate protection. In the United States, most clinicians and patients prefer the Sunday start packages, beginning on the first Sunday following menstruation. This can be easier to remember, and it usually avoids menstrual bleeding on week-ends. It is probable, but not totally certain, that even if a dominant follicle should emerge in occasional patients after a Sunday start, an LH surge and ovulation would still be prevented.[167] Some clinicians prefer to advise patients to use added protection in the first week of use.

Occasionally patients would like to postpone a menstrual period, e.g. for a wedding, holiday, or vacation. This can be easily achieved by omitting the 7-day hormone-free interval. Simply start a new package of pills the next day after finishing the series of 21 pills in the previous package. Remember, when using a 28 pill package, the patient would start a new package after using the 21 *active* pills.

The use of oral contraception shortens the duration of breastfeeding. For this reason, oral contraception is best deferred until lactation is discontinued. A good alternative is the progestin-only minipill which has no negative impact on breast milk.(See Chapters 3 and 8) The minipill has a failure rate of 3%, but when it is combined with the contraceptive action of prolactin due to lactation, nearly total protection can be achieved.

The obstetrical tradition of scheduling the postpartum visit at 6 weeks should be changed. A visit during the 3rd week allows the institution of effective contraception before ovulation resumes. After the termination of a pregnancy of less than 12 weeks, oral contraception should be started immediately. After a pregnancy of 12 or more weeks, the start of oral contraception has traditionally been delayed. The latter delay has been based on theoretical concern over an increased risk of thrombosis early in the postpartum period. This is probably no longer an issue with low dose oral contraception. We believe that oral contraception can be started immediately after a second trimester abortion or premature delivery.

There is no rationale for recommending a pill-free interval "to rest." The serious side effects are not eliminated by pill-free intervals. This practice all too often results in unwanted pregnancies.

What to do when pills are missed. *If a woman misses 1 pill,* she should take that pill as soon as she remembers and take the next pill as usual. No back-up is needed.

If she misses 2 pills in the first two weeks, she should take two pills on each of the next two days; it is unlikely that a back-up method is needed, but the official consensus is to recommend back-up for the next 7 days.

If 2 pills are missed in the third week, or if more than 2 pills are missed at any time, another form of contraception should be used as back-up immediately and for 7 days; if a Sunday starter, keep taking a pill every day until Sunday, on Sunday start a new package; if a non-Sunday starter, start a new package the same day.

Recent studies have questioned whether missing pills has an impact on contraception. One study demonstrated that after taking 7 consecutive pills, women could skip another 7 without risk of ovulation. Another study indicated that skipping 2 consecutive pills anytime between days 9 and 18 was not associated with ovulation. Studies in which women deliberately lengthen their pill-fee interval up to 11 days have failed to show signs of ovulation.[167] So far there is no evidence that moving to lower doses has had an impact on the margin of error. However, the studies have involved small numbers of women and given the large individual variation, it still is possible that some women might be at risk with a small increase in the pill-free interval. We may well prove that current recommendations are too conservative, and that a woman's chance of getting pregnant with missing pills is nearly zero. Nevertheless, this conservative advice is the safest message to convey.

Clinical Problems

Breakthrough Bleeding

A major compliance problem is breakthrough bleeding. Break-through bleeding gives rise to fears and concerns; it is aggravating, and even embarrassing. Therefore, upon starting oral contraception, patients need to be fully informed regarding breakthrough bleeding.

There are two characteristic breakthrough bleeding problems: irregular bleeding in the first few months after starting oral contraception, and unexpected bleeding after many months of use. Effort should be made to manage the bleeding problem in a way that allows the patient to remain on low dose oral contraception. *There is no evidence that indicates that the onset of bleeding is associated with decreased efficacy, no matter what oral contraceptive formulation is used, even the lowest dose products.* Indeed, in a careful study, breakthrough bleeding did not correlate with changes in the blood levels of the contraceptive steroids.[168]

The most frequently encountered breakthrough bleeding is that which occurs in the first few months of use. The incidence is greatest in the first 3 months, ranging from 10–30% in the first month to 1–10% in the third. It is best managed by encouragement and reassurance. This bleeding usually disappears by the third cycle in the majority of women. If necessary, even this early pattern of breakthrough bleeding can be treated as outlined below. It is helpful to explain to the patient that this bleeding represents tissue breakdown as the endometrium adjusts from its usual thick state to the relatively thin state allowed by the hormones in oral contraceptives.

Breakthrough bleeding which occurs after many months of oral contraceptive use is a consequence of the progestin-induced decidualization. This endometrium is shallow and tends to be fragile and prone to breakdown and asynchronous bleeding.

If bleeding occurs just before the end of the pill cycle, it can be managed by having the patient stop the pills, wait 7 days and start a new cycle. If breakthrough bleeding is prolonged or if it is aggravating for the patient, regardless of the point in the pill cycle, control of the bleeding can be achieved with a short course of exogenous estrogen. Conjugated estrogen, 1.25 mg, or estradiol, 2 mg, is administered daily for 7 days when the bleeding is present, no matter where the patient is in her pill cycle. The patient continues to adhere to the schedule of pill taking. Usually one course of estrogen solves the problem, and recurrence of bleeding is unusual (but if it does recur, another 7-day course of estrogen is effective).

Responding to irregular bleeding by having the patient take 2 or 3 pills is not effective. The progestin component of the pill will always dominate, hence doubling the number of pills will also double the progestational impact and its decidualizing, atrophic effect on the endometrium. The addition of extra estrogen while keeping the progestin dose unchanged is logical and effective. This allows the patient to remain on the low dose formulation with its advantage of greater safety. Breakthrough bleeding, in our view, is not sufficient reason to expose patients to the increased risks associated with higher dose oral contraceptives. Any bleeding which is not handled by this routine requires investigation for the presence of pathology.

There is no evidence that any specific formulation is significantly superior to any other in terms of the rate of breakthrough bleeding. Clinicians often become impressed that switching to another specific product effectively stops the breakthrough bleeding. It is more likely that the passage of time is the responsible factor, and bleeding would have stopped regardless of switching and regardless of product.

Amenorrhea

With low dose pills, the estrogen content is not sufficient in some women to stimulate endometrial growth. The progestational effect dominates to such a degree that a shallow atrophic endometrium is produced, lacking sufficient tissue to yield withdrawal bleeding. It should be emphasized that permanent atrophy of the endometrium does not occur, and resumption of normal ovarian function will restore endometrial growth and development. Indeed, there is no harmful, permanent consequence of developing amenorrhea while on oral contraception.

The major problem with amenorrhea while on oral contraception is the anxiety produced in both patient and clinician because the lack of bleeding may be a sign of pregnancy. The patient is anxious because of the uncertainty regarding pregnancy, and the clinician is anxious because of the medical-legal concerns stemming from the old studies which indicated an increased risk of congenital abnormalities among the offspring of women who inadvertently used oral contraception in early pregnancy. We reviewed this problem earlier, and emphatically stated that there is no association between oral contraception and an increased risk of congenital malformation, and there is no increased risk of having abnormal children.

The incidence of amenorrhea in the first year of use with low dose oral contraception is less than 1%. This incidence increases with duration, reaching perhaps 5% after several years of use. It is important to alert patients upon starting oral contraception that diminished bleeding and possibly no bleeding may ensue.

Amenorrhea is a difficult management problem. A pregnancy test will allow reliable assessment for the presence of pregnancy even at this early stage. However, routine, repeated use of such testing is expensive and annoying, and may lead to discontinuation of oral contraception. *A simple test for pregnancy is to assess the basal body temperature during the END of the pill-free week; a basal body temperature less than 98 degrees is inconsistent with pregnancy and oral contraception can be continued.*

Many women are reassured with an understanding of why there is no bleeding and are able to continue on the pill despite the amenorrhea. Some women cannot reconcile themselves to a lack of bleeding, and this is an indication for trying other formulations (a practice unsupported by any clinical trials, and therefore, the expectations are uncertain). But again, this problem does not warrant exposing patients to the greater risks of major side effects associated with higher dose products.

Some clinicians have observed that the addition of extra estrogen for 1 month (1.25 mg conjugated estrogen or 2 mg estradiol daily throughout the 21 days while taking the oral contraceptive) will rejuvenate the endometrium, and withdrawal bleeding will resume, persisting for many months.

Weight Gain

The complaint of weight gain is frequently cited as a major problem with compliance. Yet studies of the low dose preparations fail to demonstrate a significant weight gain with oral contraception, and no major differences among the various products. This is obviously a problem of perception. The clinician has to carefully reinforce the lack of association between low dose oral contraceptives and weight gain and focus the patient on the real culprit: diet and level of exercise.

Acne

Regardless of which preparation is used, low dose oral contraceptives improve acne. The low progestin doses (including levonorgestrel formulations) currently used are insufficient to stimulate this androgenic response.

Ovarian Cysts

Anecdotal reports suggested that ovarian cysts are encountered more frequently and suppress less easily with multiphasic formulations. This observation failed to withstand careful scrutiny.[169] Functional ovarian cysts occur less frequently in women on oral contraception (although this beneficial effect is not seen with the progestin-only minipill).[170] But the risk of such cysts is not eliminated entirely, and therefore, clinicians can encounter such cysts in patients taking any of the oral contraceptive formulations.

Drugs Which Affect Efficacy

There are many anecdotal reports of patients who conceived on oral contraceptives while taking antibiotics. There is little evidence, however, that antibiotics such as ampicillin, metronidazole, quinolone, and tetracycline, which reduce the bacterial flora of the gastrointestinal tract, affect oral contraceptive efficacy. Studies indicate that while antibiotics can alter the excretion of contraceptive steroids, plasma levels are unchanged, and there is no evidence of ovulation.[171,172]

There is good reason to believe that drugs which stimulate the liver's metabolic capacity can affect oral contraceptive efficacy. On the other hand, a search of a large database failed to discover any evidence that lower dose oral contraceptives are more likely to fail or to have more drug interaction problems when other drugs are used.[173]

To be cautious, patients on medications that affect liver metabolism should choose an alternative contraceptive. These drugs are as follows:

Rifampin
Phenobarbital
Phenytoin (Dilantin)
Primidone (Mysoline)
Carbamazepine (Tegretol)

Other Drug Interactions

Although not extensively documented, there is reason to believe that oral contraceptives potentiate the action of diazepam (Valium), chlordiazepoxide (Librium), tricyclic antidepressants, and theophylline.[174–176] Thus, lower doses of these agents may be effective in oral contraceptive users. Because of an influence on clearance rates, oral contraceptive users may require larger doses of acetaminophen and aspirin.[177,178]

Migraine Headaches

True migraine headaches are more common in women, while tension headaches occur equally in men and women. There have been no well-done studies to determine the impact of oral contraception on migraine headaches. Patients may report that their headaches are worse, or better.

Studies with high dose pills indicated that migraine headaches were linked to a risk of stroke. There is reason to believe that the combination of good patient screening and the use of low dose oral contraception has virtually eliminated the risk of stroke. Nevertheless, because of the seriousness of this potential complication, the onset of visual symptoms or severe headaches requires a serious response. Certainly if the patient is at a higher dose, a move to a low dose formulation often relieves the symptom. Switching to a different brand is worthwhile, if only to evoke a placebo response. True vascular headaches are an indication to discontinue oral contraception.

Clues to severe vascular headaches:

- Headaches which last a long time.
- Dizziness, nausea, or vomiting with headaches.
- Scotomata or blurred vision.
- Episodes of blindness.
- Unilateral, unremitting headaches.
- Headaches which continue despite medication.

In some women, a relationship exists between their fluctuating hormone levels during a menstrual cycle and migraine headaches, with the onset of headaches characteristically coinciding with menses. We have had personal success (anecdotal to be sure) alleviating headaches by eliminating the menstrual cycle, either with the use of daily oral contraceptives or the daily administration of a progestational agent (such as 10 mg medroxyprogesterone acetate). Some women with migraine headaches have extremely gratifying responses.

Summary: OC Use and Medical Problems

Gestational Diabetes. There is no contraindication to oral contraceptive use following gestational diabetes.

Diabetes Mellitus. Oral contraception can be used by diabetic women less than 35 years old, who do not smoke and are otherwise healthy (especially an absence of diabetic vascular complications).

Hypertension. Low dose oral contraception can be used in women less than age 35 years old with hypertension controlled by medication, and who are otherwise healthy and do not smoke.

Pregnancy-Induced Hypertension. Women with pregnancy-induced hypertension can use oral contraception as soon as the blood pressure is normal in the postpartum period.

Gallbladder Disease. Oral contraception use may precipitate a symptomatic attack in women known to have stones or a positive history for gallbladder disease, and therefore, should either be used very cautiously or not at all.

Obesity. An obese woman who is otherwise healthy can use low dose oral contraception.

Hepatic Disease. Oral contraception can be utilized when liver function tests return to normal. Follow-up liver function tests should be obtained after 2–3 months of use.

Seizure Disorders. There is no impact of oral contraceptives on pattern or frequency of seizures; anticonvulsant doses can decrease. The concern is that anticonvulsant-induced hepatic enzyme activity can increase the risk of contraceptive failure. Some clinicians advocate the use of higher dose (50 µg estrogen) products.

Mitral Valve Prolapse. Oral contraception use is limited to patients who have only the echocardiographic diagnosis and are free of the clinical findings of mitral regurgitation.

Systemic Lupus Erythematosus. Oral contraceptive use can excacerbate systemic lupus erythematous, and the vascular disease associated with lupus represents a contraindication to estrogen-containing oral contraceptives.[179] The progestin-only methods can be considered.

Migraine Headaches. Low dose oral contraception can be tried with careful surveillance. Daily administration can prevent menstrual migraine headaches.

Sickle Cell Disease. Patients with sickle cell trait can use oral contraception. The risk of thrombosis in women with sickle cell disease or sickle C diseases is theoretical (and medical-legal). We believe effective protection against pregnancy in these patients warrants the use of low dose oral contraception.

Benign Breast Disease. Benign breast disease is not a contraindication for oral contraception; with 2 years of use, the condition can improve.

Congenital Heart Disease or Valvular Heart Disease. Oral contraception is contraindicated only if there is marginal cardiac reserve or a condition which predisposes to thrombosis.

Hyperlipidemia. Because low dose oral contraceptives have negligible impact on the lipoprotein profile, hyperlipidemia is not a contraindication, with the exception of very high levels of triglycerides (which can be made worse by oral contraception). Of course, if vascular disease is already present, oral contraception should be avoided.

81

Depression. Low dose oral contraceptives have minimal, if any, impact on mood.

Smoking. Oral contraception is absolutely contraindicated in smokers over the age of 35. In patients 35 years old and less, heavy smoking (15 or more cigarettes per day) is a relative contraindication. The data indicate no increased risk of dying of a cardiovascular event in smokers under the age of 30. A ex-smoker should be regarded as a nonsmoker. Risk is only linked to active smoking.

Pituitary Prolactin-Secreting Adenomas. Low dose oral contraception can be used in the presence of microadenomas.

Infectious Mononucleosis. Oral contraception can be used as long as liver function tests are normal.

Ulcerative Colitis. There is no association between oral contraception and ulcerative colitis; women with this problem can use oral contraceptives.[180] Oral contraceptives are absorbed mainly in the small bowel.

An Alternative Route of Administration

Occasionally a situation may be encountered when an alternative to oral administration of contraceptive pills is required. For example, patients receiving chemotherapy can either have significant nausea and vomiting, or mucocitis, both of which would prevent oral drug administration. The low-dose oral contraceptives can be administered vaginally. However, two pills must be placed high in the vagina daily in order to produce contraceptive steroid blood levels comparable to the oral administration of one pill.[181,182]

Noncontraceptive Benefits

The noncontraceptive benefits of oral contraception can be grouped into two main categories: benefits which incidentally accrue when oral contraception is specifically utilized for contraceptive purposes, and benefits which result from the use of oral contraceptives to treat problems and disorders.

The noncontraceptive incidental benefits can be listed as follows:

> Effective Contraception.
>> • less need for therapeutic abortion.
>> • less need for surgical sterilization.
>
> Less Endometrial Cancer.
> Less Ovarian Cancer.
> Less Benign Breast Disease.
> Fewer Ovarian Cysts.
> Fewer Uterine Fibroids.
> Fewer Ectopic Pregnancies.
> More Regular Menses.
>> • less flow.
>> • less dysmenorrhea.
>> • less anemia.
>
> Less Salpingitis.
> Less Rheumatoid Arthritis.
> Increased Bone Density.
> Probably Less Endometriosis.
> Possibly Protection Against Atherosclerosis.

Many of these benefits have been previously discussed. Protection against pelvic inflammatory disease is especially noteworthy, and a major contribution to not only preservation of fertility but to lower health care costs. Also important is the prevention of ectopic pregnancies. Ectopic pregnancies have increased in incidence (undoubtedly due to an increase in STDs) and represent a major cost for our society, and a threat to both fertility and life for individual patients.

Of course, prevention of benign and malignant neoplasia is an outstanding feature of oral contraception. A 40% reduction in ovarian cancer and a 50% reduction in endometrial cancer represent substantial protection. The OFPA study has documented in long-term users a 31% reduction in uterine leiomyomata, and in current users a 78% reduction in corpus luteum cysts, and a 49% reduction in functional ovarian cysts.[164,170] The result is a net reduction in surgical procedures and lives saved. Oral contraceptive use decreases the incidence of benign breast disease diagnosed clinically, as well as fibrocystic disease and fibroadenomas diagnosed by biopsy.

The low dose contraceptives are as effective as higher dose preparations in reducing the prevalence and severity of dysmenorrhea.[183] Experience has proven that low dose oral contraceptives effectively provide the benefits associated with a reduction in menstrual flow. Previous use of oral contraception is associated with a lower incidence of endometriosis,[184] but the impact on bone is less certain. Although some studies have documented an increase in vertebral bone density with exposure to oral contraception, others have not.[185,186] On the other hand, an Austrian study concluded that osteoporosis occurs later and is less frequent in women who have used long-term oral contraception.[187] A cross-sectional study of postmenopausal women concluded that prior use of oral contraception is associated with higher levels of bone density and that the degree of protection is related to duration of exposure.[188] As women who have had the opportunity to use oral contraception are just now entering the postmenopausal years, it will be several years before this question is answered.

The literature on rheumatoid arthritis has been controversial, with studies in Europe finding evidence of protection and studies in North America failing to demonstrate such an effect.[189,190] An excellent Danish case-control study was designed to answer criticisms of short-comings in the previous literature.[191] Ever use of oral contraception reduced the relative risk of rheumatoid arthritis by 60%, and the strongest protection was present in women with a positive family history. A meta-analysis concluded that the evidence consistently indicated a protective effect, but that rather than preventing the development of rheumatoid arthritis, oral contraception may modify the course of disease, inhibiting progression of the disease.[192]

Oral contraceptives are frequently utilized to manage the following problems and disorders:

Definitely Beneficial:
- dysfunctional uterine bleeding.
- dysmenorrhea.
- mittelschmerz.
- endometriosis prophylaxis.
- acne and hirsutism.
- hormone replacement for hypothalamic amenorrhea.
- prevention of menstrual porphyria.

Probably Beneficial:
- functional ovarian cysts.
- premenstrual syndrome.
- control of bleeding (dyscrasias, anovulation).

85

Oral contraceptives have been a cornerstone for the treatment of anovulatory, dysfunctional uterine bleeding. For patients who need effective contraception, oral contraceptives are a good choice to provide hormone replacement to amenorrheic patients, as well as to treat dysmenorrhea. Oral contraceptives are also a good choice to provide prophylaxis against the recurrence of endometriosis in a woman who has already undergone more vigorous treatment with surgery or the GnRH analogues. In this instance, we recommend that the oral contraceptives be taken daily, with no break, and no withdrawal bleeding.

The low dose oral contraceptives are effective in treating acne and hirsutism. Suppression of free testosterone levels is comparable to that achieved with higher dosage.[193] The beneficial clinical effect is the same with low dose preparations containing levonorgestrel, previously recognized to cause acne at high dosage.[194]

Oral contraceptives have long been used to speed the resolution of ovarian cysts, but the efficacy of this treatment has never been studied. In a small study, 24 patients who had persistent cysts after exogenous gonadotropin treatment were randomized to receive an oral contraceptive or expectant management.[195] No advantage for the contraceptive treatment could be demonstrated. The cysts resolved completely and equally fast in both groups. Of course, these were functional cysts secondary to ovulation induction, and this experience may not apply to spontaneously appearing cysts. We continue to treat patients with ovarian simple cysts with oral contraceptives, even though we recognize that the efficacy of this treatment has never been proven. Oral contraception does provide protection in women who repetitively form ovarian cysts.

Conclusion. Oral contraceptives are associated with a collection of effects which yield an overall improvement in individual health. From a public health point of view, the combined impact leads to a decrease in the cost of health care. For both the individual and the public health, these impacts are especially significant in older women. These considerations allow the clinician to present oral contraception with a very positive attitude, an approach which makes an important contribution to a patient's ability to make appropriate health choices.

Compliance: Failure or Success?

Despite the fact that oral contraception is highly effective, hundreds of thousands of unintended pregnancies occur each year in the United States because of the failure of oral contraception. World-wide, literally millions of unintended pregnancies result from poor compliance. In general, young, unmarried, poor, and minority women are more likely to have failures, reaching rates of 10–20%.[196] Overall, the failure rate with actual use ranges from 3 to 6%. This difference between the theoretical efficacy and actual use reflects compliance and noncompliance. Noncompliance includes a wide variety of behavior: failure to fill the initial prescription, failure to continue on the medication, and incorrectly taking oral contraception. Compliance is an area in which personal behavior, biology, and pharmacology come together. Oral contraceptive compliance reflects the interaction of these influences.

There are 3 major factors that affect compliance:

1. Fears and concerns regarding cancer, cardiovascular disease, and the impact of oral contraception on future fertility.
2. The experience of side effects such as breakthrough bleeding and amenorrhea, and perceived experience of "minor" problems such as headaches, nausea, and weight gain.
3. Non-medical issues such as inadequate instructions on pill-taking, complicated pill packaging, and difficulties arising from the patient package insert.

The information in this chapter is the foundation for good compliance, but the clinician must go beyond the presentation of information and develop an effective means of communicating that information. We recommend the following approach to the clinician-patient encounter as one way to improve compliance with oral contraception.

1. Explain how oral contraception works.
2. Review briefly the risks and benefits of oral contraception, but be careful to put the risks in proper perspective, and to emphasize the safety and noncontraceptive benefits of low dose oral contraceptives.
3. Show and demonstrate to the patient the package of pills she will use.

4. Explain how to take the pills:
   • When to start.
   • To develop a daily routine to avoid missing pills.
   • What to do if pills are missed.
5. Review the side effects that can affect compliance: amenorrhea, breakthrough bleeding, headaches, weight gain, nausea, etc., and what to do if one or more occurs.
6. Explain the warning signs of potential problems: abdominal or chest pain, trouble breathing, severe headaches, visual problems, leg pain or swelling.
7. Ask the patient to be sure to call if another clinician prescribes other medications.
8. Ask the patient to repeat critical information to make sure she understands what has been said. Ask if the patient has any questions.
9. Schedule a return appointment in 2–3 months to review understanding and address fears and concerns.
10. Make sure a line of communication is open to a clinician or office personnel. Ask the patient to call for any problem or concern before she stops taking the oral contraceptives.

References

1. Goldzieher JW, Hormonal Contraception—whence, how, and whither? in Givens J, editor, *Clinical Uses of Steroids,* Yearbook, Chicago, 1980, pp 31–43.

2. Medvei VC, *A History of Endocrinology,* MTB Press, Hingham, Massachusetts, 1982.

3. Pincus, G, *The Control of Fertility,* Academic Press, New York, 1965.

4. Goldzieher JW, Selected aspects of the pharmacokinetics and metabolism of ethinyl estrogens and their clinical implications, Am J Obstet Gynecol 163:318, 1990.

5. Stanczyk FZ, Roy S, Metabolism of levonorgestrel, norethindrone, and structurally related contraceptive steroids, Contraception 42:67, 1990.

6. Edgren RA, Progestagens, in Givens J, editor, *Clinical Uses of Steroids,* Yearbook, Chicago, 1980, pp 1–29.

7. Trussell J, Hatcher RA, Cates W Jr, Stewart FH, Kost K, Contraceptive failure in the United States: An update, Stud Fam Plann 21:51, 1990.

8. Royal College of General Practitioners, *Oral Contraceptives and Health,* Pitman Publishing, New York, 1974.

9. Royal College of General Practitioners, Oral contraception study: Mortality among oral contraceptive users, Lancet ii:727, 1977.

10. Royal College of General Practitioners, Oral contraceptive study: Oral contraceptives, venous thrombosis, and varicose veins, J Roy Coll Gen Pract 28:393, 1978.

11. Royal College of General Practitioners Oral Contraceptive Study, Further analyses of mortality in oral contraceptive users, Lancet i:541, 1981.

88

12. Royal College of General Practitioners Oral Contraceptive Study, Incidence of arterial disease among oral contraceptive users, J Roy Coll Gen Pract 33:75, 1983.

13. Vessey MP, McPherson K, Johnson B, Mortality among women participating in the Oxford/Family Planning Association contraceptive study, Lancet ii:731, 1977.

14. Vessey MP, McPherson K, Yeates D, Mortality in oral contraceptive users, Lancet i:549, 1981.

15. Vessey MP, Lawless M, Yeates D, Oral Contraceptives and stroke: Findings in a large prospective study, Br Med J 289:530, 1984.

16. Ramcharan S, Pellegrin FA, Ray RM, Hsu J-P, The Walnut Creek Contraceptive Drug Study. A prospective study of the side effects of oral contraceptives, J Reprod Med 25:360,366, 1980.

17. Ory HW, Association between oral contraceptives and myocardial infarction, JAMA 237:2619, 1977.

18. Shapiro S, Slone D, Rosenberg L, Kaufman DW, Stolley PD, Miettinen OS, Oral contraceptive use in relation to myocardial infarction, Lancet i:743, 1979.

19. Hennekens CH, Evans D, Peto R, Oral contraceptive use, cigarette smoking and myocardial infarction, Br J Fam Plann 5:66, 1979.

20. Rosenberg L, Hennekens CH, Rosner B, Belanger C, Rothman KH, Speizer FE, Oral contraceptive use in relation to nonfatal myocardial infarction, Am J Epidemiol 11:59, 1980.

21. Meade TW, Greenburg G, Thompson SG, Progestogens and cardiovascular reactions associated with oral contraceptives and a comparison of the safety of 50- and 30- µg estrogen preparations, Br Med J 280:1157, 1980.

22. Kay CR, The happiness pill, J Roy Coll Gen Pract 30:8, 1980.

69

23. Collaborative Group for the Study of Stroke in Young Women, Oral contraceptives and stroke in young women, JAMA 231:718, 1975.

24. Porter JB, Hershel J, Walker AM, Mortality among oral contraceptive users, Obstet Gynecol 70:29, 1987.

25. Tietze C, The pill and mortality from cardiovascular disease: Another look, Fam Plann Perspect 11:80, 1979.

26. Belsey MA, Russel Y, Kinnear K, Cardiovascular disease and oral contraceptives: A reappraisal of vital statistics data, Fam Plann Perspect 11:84, 1979.

27. Vessey MP, Villard-Mackintosh I, McPherson K, Yeates D, Mortality among oral contraceptive users: 20 year follow up of women in a cohort study, Br Med J 299:1487, 1989.

28. Bottinger LE, Boman G, Eklund G, Westerholm B, Oral contraceptives and thromboembolic disease: Effects of lowering oestrogen content, Lancet i:1097, 1980.

29. Gerstman BB, Piper JM, Tomita DK, Ferguson WJ, Stadel BV, Lundin FE, Oral contraceptive estrogen dose and the risk of deep venous thromboembolic disease, Am J Epidemiol 133:32, 1991.

30. Bonnar J, Coagulation effects of oral contraception, Am J Obstet Gynecol 157:1042, 1987.

31. Inauen W, Stocker G, Haeberli A, Straub PW, Effects of low and high dose oral contraceptives on blood coagulation and thrombogenesis induced by vascular endothelium exposed to flowing human blood, Contraception 43:435, 1991.

32. Daly L, Bonnar J, Comparative studies of 30 μg ethinyl estradiol combined with gestodene and desogestrel on blood coagulation, fibrinolysis, and platelets, Am J Obstet Gynecol 163:430, 1990.

33. Abbate R, Pinto S, Rostagno C, Bruni V, Rosati D, Mariani G, Effects of long-term gestodene-containing oral contraceptive administration on hemostasis, Am J Obstet Gynecol 163:424, 1990.

34. Jespersen J, Petersen KR, Skouby SO, Effects of newer oral contraceptives on the inhibition of coagulation and fibrinolysis in relation to dosage and type of steroid, Am J Obstet Gynecol 163:396, 1990.

35. Stampfer MJ, Willett WC, Colditz GA, Speizer FE, Hennekens CH, Past use of oral contraceptives and cardiovascular disease: A meta-analysis in the context of the Nurses' Health Study, Am J Obstet Gynecol 163:285, 1990.

36. Rosenberg L, Palmer JR, Lesko SM, Shapiro S, Oral contraceptive use and the risk of myocardial infarction, Am J Epidemiol 131:1009, 1990.

37. Croft P, Hannaford PC, Risk factors for acute myocardial infarction in women: Evidence from the Royal College of General Practitioners' oral contraception study, Br Med J 298:165, 1989.

38. Wahl P, Walden C, Knopp R, Hoover J, Wallace R, Heiss G, Refkind B, Effect of estrogen/progestin potency on lipid/lipoprotein cholesterol, New Engl J Med 308:862, 1983.

49. Burkman RT, Robinson JC, Kruszon-Moran D, Kimball AW, Kwiterovich P, Burford RG, Lipid and lipoprotein changes associated with oral contraceptive use: A randomized clinical trial, Obstet Gynecol 71:33, 1988.

40. Patsch W, Brown SA, Grotto AM Jr, Young RL, The effect of triphasic oral contraceptives on plasma lipids and lipoproteins, Am J Obstet Gynecol 161:1396, 1989.

41. Gevers Leuven JA, Dersjant-Roorda MC, Helmerhorst FM, de Boer R, Neymeyer-Leloux A, Havekes L, Estrogenic effect of gestodene-desogestrel-containing oral contraceptives on lipoprotein metabolism, Am J Obstet Gynecol 163:358, 1990.

42. Kloosterboer HJ, Rekers H, Effects of three combined oral contraceptive preparations containing desogestrel plus ethinyl estradiol on lipid metabolism in comparison with two levonorgestrel preparations, Am J Obstet Gynecol 163:370, 1990.

43. Notelovitz M, Feldmand EB, Gillespy M, Gudat J, Lipid and lipoprotein changes in women taking low-dose, triphasic oral contraceptives: A controlled, comparative, 12-month clinical trial, Am J Obstet Gynecol 160:1269, 1989.

44. Engel JH, Engel E, Lichtlen PR, Coronary atherosclerosis and myocardial infarction in young women—role of oral contraceptives, Eur Heart J 4:1, 1983.

45. Jugdutt BI, Stevens GF, Zacks DJ, Lee SJK, Taylor RF, Myocardial infarction, oral contraception, cigarette smoking, and coronary artery spasm in young women, Am Heart J 106:757, 1983.

46. Croft P, Hannaford PC, Risk factors for acute myocardial infarction in women, Br Med J 298:674, 1989.

47. Adams MR, Clarkson TB, Koritnik DR, Nash HA, Contraceptive steroids and coronary artery atherosclerosis in cynomolgus macaques, Fertil Steril 47:1010, 1987.

48. Clarkson TB, Adams MR, Kaplan JR, Shively CA, Koritnik DR, From menarche to menoause: Coronary artery atherosclerosis and protection in cynomolgus monkeys, Am J Obst Gynecol 160:1280, 1989.

49. Clarkson TB, Shively CA, Morgan TM, Koritnik DR, Adams MR, Kaplan JR, Oral contraceptives and coronary artery atherosclerosis of cynomolgus monkeys, Obstet Gynecol 75:217, 1990.

50. Kushwaha RS, Hazzard WR, Exogenous estrogens attenuate dietary hypercholesterolemia and atherosclerosis in the rabbit, Metabolism 30:57, 1981.

51. Hough JL, Zilversmit DB, Effect of 17 beta estradiol on aortic cholesterol content and metabolism in cholesterol-fed rabbits, Arteriosclerosis 6:57, 1986.

52. Henriksson P, Stamberger M, Eriksson M, Rudling M, Diczfulusy U, Berglund L, Angelin B, Oestrogen-induced changes in lipoprotein metabolism: Role in prevention of atherosclerosis in the cholesterol-fed rabbit, Eur J Clin Invest 19:395, 1989.

53. Hirvonen E, Heikkila-Idanpaan J, Cardiovascular death among women under 40 years of age using low-estrogen oral contraceptives and intrauterine devices in Finland from 1975 to 1984, Am J Obstet Gynecol 163:281, 1990.

54. Mant D, Villard-Mackintosh L, Vessey MP, Yeates D, Myocardial infarction and angina pectoris in young women, J Epidemiol Community Health 41:215, 1987.

55. Khaw K-T, Peart WS, Blood pressure and contraceptive use, Br Med J 285:403, 1982.

56. Wilson E, Cruickshank I, McMaster M, Weir RJ, A prospective controlled study of the effect on blood pressure of contraceptive preparations containing different types and dosages of progestogen, Br J Obstet Gynaecol 91:1254, 1984.

57. Kovacs L, Bartfai G, Apro G, Annus J, Bulpitt C, Belsey E, Pinol A, The effect of the contraceptive pill on blood pressure: A randomized controlled trial of three progestogen-oestrogen combinations in Szeged, Hungary, Contraception 33:69, 1986.

58. Pritchard JA, Pritchard SA, Blood pressure response to estrogen-progestin oral contraceptives after pregnancy-induced hypertension, Am J Obstet Gynecol 129:733, 1977.

59. Gaspard UJ, Lefebvre PJ, Clinical aspects of the relationship between oral contraceptives, abnormalities in carbohydrate metabolism, and the development of cardiovascular disease, Am J Obstet Gynecol 163:334, 1990.

93

60. Bowes WA, Katta LR, Droegemueller W, Braight TG, Triphasic randomized clinical trial: Comparison of effects on carbohydrate metabolism, Am J Obstet Gynecol 161:1402, 1989.

61. van der Vange N, Kloosterboer HJ, Haspels AA, Effect of seven low-dose combined oral contraceptive preparations on carbohydrate metabolism, Am J Obstet Gynecol 156:918, 1987.

62. Godsland IF, Crook D, Simpson R, Proudler T, Gelton C, Lees B, Anyaoku V, Devenport M, Wynn V, The effects of different formulations of oral contraceptive agents on lipid and carbohydrate metabolism, New Engl J Med 323:1375, 1990.

63. Duffy TJ, Ray R, Oral contraceptive use: Prospective follow-up of women with suspected glucose intolerance, Contraception 30:197, 1984.

64. Hannaford PC, Kay CR, Oral contraceptives and diabetes mellitus, Br Med J 299:315, 1989.

65. Kung AWC, Ma JTC, Wong VCW, Li DFH, Ng MMT, Wang CCL, Lam KSL, Young RTT, Ma HK, Glucose and lipid metabolism with triphasic oral contraceptives in women with history of gestational diabetes, Contraception 35:257, 1987.

66. Skouby SO, Kuhl C, Molsted-Pedersen L, Petersen K, Christensen MS, Triphasic oral contraception: Metabolic effects in normal women and those with previous gestational diabetes, Am J Obstet Gynecol 153:495, 1985.

67. Skouby SO, Andersen O, Saurbrey N, Kuhl C, Oral contraception and insulin sensitivity: *In vivo* assessment in normal women and women with previous gestational diabetes, J Clin Endocrinol Metab 64:519, 1987.

68. Kjos SL, Shoupe D, Douyan S, Friedman RL, Bernstein GS, Mestman JH, Mishell DR Jr, Effect of low-dose oral contraceptives on carbohydrate and lipid metabolism in women with recent gestational diabetes: Results of a controlled, randomized, prospective study, Am J Obstet Gynecol 163:1822, 1990.

69. Royal College of General Practitioners' Oral Contraception Study, Oral contraceptives and gallbladder disease, Lancet ii:957, 1982.

70. Bennion LJ, Ginsberg RL, Garnick MB, Bennett PH, Effects of oral contraceptives on the gallbladder bile of normal women, New Engl J Med 294:189, 1976.

71. Hulting A-L, Werner S, Hagenfeldt K, Oral contraceptives do not promote the development or growth of prolactinomas, Contraception 27:69, 1983.

72. The Cancer and Steroid Hormone Study of the CDC and NICHD, Combination oral contraceptive use and the risk of endometrial cancer, JAMA 257:796, 1987.

73. The Cancer and Steroid Hormone Study of the CDC and NICHD, The reduction in risk of ovarian cancer associated with oral-contraceptive use, New Engl J Med 316:650, 1987.

74. Brinton LA, Oral contraceptives and cervical neoplasia, Contraception 43:581, 1991.

75. Irwin KL, Rosero-Bixby L, Oberle MW, Lee NC, Whatley AS, Fortney JA, Bonhomme MG, Oral contraceptives and cervical cancer risk in Costa Rica: Detection bias or causal association? JAMA 259:59, 1988.

76. Brinton LA, Reeves WC, Brenes MM, Herrero R, De Britton RC, Gaitan E, Tenorio F, Garcia M, Rawls WE, Oral contraceptive use and risk of invasive cervical cancer, Int J Epidemiol 19:4, 1990.

77. Neuberger J, Forman D, Doll R, Williams R, Oral contraceptives and hepatocellular carcinoma, Br Med J 292:1355, 1986.

78. Palmer JR, Rosenberg L, Kaufman DW, Warshauer ME, Stolley P, Shapiro S, Oral contraceptive use and liver cancer, Am J Epidemiol 130:878, 1989.

79. WHO Collaborative Study of Neoplasia and Steroid Contraceptives, Combined oral contraceptives and liver cancer, Int J Cancer 43:254, 1989.

80. Brinton LA, Vessey MP, Flavel R, Yeates D, Risk factors for benign breast disease, Am J Epidemiol 113:203, 1981.

81. Vessey M, Baron J, Doll R, McPherson K, Yeates D, Oral contraceptives and breast cancer: Final report of an epidemiological study, Br J Cancer 47:455, 1982.

82. Vessey M, McPherson K, Villard-Mackintosh L, Yeates D, Oral contraceptives and breast cancer: Latest findings in a large cohort study, Br J Cancer 59:613, 1989.

83. Romieu I, Willett WC, Colditz GA, Stampfer MJ, Rosner B, Hennekens, CH, Speizer FE, Prospective study of oral contraceptive use and risk of breast cancer in women, JNCI 81:1313, 1989.

84. La Vecchia C, Decarli A, Fasoli M, Franceschi S, Gentile A, Negri E, Parazzini F, Tognomi G, Oral contraceptives and cancers of the breast and of the female genital tract. Interim results from a case-control study, Br J Cancer 54:311, 1986.

85. Meirik O, Dami H, Christoffersen T, Lund E, Bergstrom R, Bergsjo P, Oral contraceptive use and breast cancer in young women, Lancet ii:650, 1986.

86. Kay CR, Hannaford PC, Breast cancer and the pill—further report from the Royal College of General Practitioners' oral contraceptive study, Br J Cancer 58:675, 1988.

87. Miller DR, Rosenberg L, Kaufman DW, Stolley P, Warshauer ME, Shapiro S, Breast cancer before age 45 and oral contraceptive use: New findings, Am J Epidemiol 129:269, 1989.

88. UK National Case-Control Study Group, Oral contraceptive use and breast cancer risk in young women, Lancet i:973, 1989.

89. WHO Collaborative Study of Neoplasia and Steroid Contraceptives, Breast cancer and combined oral contraceptives: Results from a multinational study, Br J Cancer 61:110, 1990.

90. McPherson K, Neil A, Vessey MP, Oral contraceptives and breast cancer, Lancet ii:414, 1983.

91. Hennekens CH, Speizer FE, Lipnik RJ, Rosner B, Bain C, Belanger C, Stampfer MJ, Willett W, Peto R, Case-control study of oral contraceptive use and breast cancer, JNCI 72:39, 1984.

92. Rosenberg L, Miller DR, Kaufman DW, Helmrich SP, Stolley PD, Schoffenfeld D, Shapiro S, Breast cancer and oral contraceptive use, Am J Epidemiol 119:167, 1984.

93. Stadel BV, Rubin GL, Webster LA, Schlesselman JJ, Wingo PA, Oral contraceptives and breast cancer in young women, Lancet ii:970, 1985.

94. Paul C, Skegg DCG, Spears GFS, Kaldor JM, Oral contraceptives and breast cancer: A national study, Br Med J 293:723, 1986.

95. McPherson K, Vessey MP, Neil A, Doll R, Jones L, Roberts M, Early oral contraceptive use and breast cancer: Results of another case-control study, Br J Cancer 56:653, 1987.

96. Stadel BV, Lai SL, Oral contraceptives and premenopausal breast cancer in nulliparous women, Contraception 38:287, 1988.

97. Stanford JL, Brinton LA, Hoover RN, Oral contraceptives and breast cancer: Results from an expanded case-control study, Br J Cancer 60:375, 1989.

98. Schildkraut JM, Hulka BS, Wilkinson WE, Oral contraceptives and breast cancer: A case-control study with hospital and community controls, Obstet Gynecol 76:395, 1990.

99. Lipnick RJ, Buring JE, Hennekens CH, Rosner B, Willett W, Bain C, Stampfer MJ, Colditz GA, Peto R, Speizer FE, Oral contraceptives and breast cancer: A prospective cohort study, JAMA 255:58, 1986.

100. Pike MC, Krailo MD, Henderson BE, Duke A, Roy S, Breast cancer in young women and use of oral contraceptives: Possible modifying effect of formulation and age at use, Lancet ii:926, 1983.

101. Miller DR, Rosenberg L, Kaufman DW, Schottenfeld D, Stolley PD, Shapiro S, Breast cancer risk in relation to early oral contraceptive use, Obstet Gynecol 68:863, 1986.

102. Cancer and Steroid Hormone Study, CDC and NICHD, Oral contraceptive use and the risk of breast cancer, New Engl J Med 315:405, 1986.

103. Murray P, Schlesselman JJ, Stadel BV, Shenghan L, Oral contraceptives and breast cancer risk in women with a family history of breast cancer, Am J Obstet Gynecol 73:977, 1989.

104. Schlesselman JJ, Stadel BV, Murray P, Shenghan L, Breast cancer risk in relation to type of estrogen contained in oral contraceptives, Contraception 36:595, 1987.

105. Schlesselman JJ, Stadel BV, Murray P, Lai S, Breast cancer in relation to early use of oral contracpetives. No evidence of a latent effect, JAMA 259:1828, 1988.

106. Wingo PA, Lee NC, Ory HW, Beral V, Peterson HB, Rhodes P, Age-specific differences in the relationship between oral contraceptive use and breast cancer, Obstet Gynecol 78:161, 1991.

107. Paul C, Skegg DCG, Spears GFS, Oral contraceptives and risk of breast cancer, Int J Cancer 46:366, 1990

108. National Cancer Institute, Annual cancer statistics review, including cancer trends: 1950–1985, National Institutes of Health, Bethesda, 1989.

109. Stadel BV, Schlesselman JJ, Oral contraceptive use and the risk of breast cancer in women with a "prior" history of benign breast disease, Am J Epidemiol 123:373, 1986.

110. Green A, Oral contraceptives and skin neoplasia, Contraception 43:653, 1991.

111. Hannaford PC, Villard-Mackintosh L, Vessey MP, Kay CR, Oral contraceptives and malignant melanoma, Br J Cancer 63:430, 1991.

112. Milne R, Vessey M, The association of oral contraception with kidney cancer, colon cancer, gallbladder cancer (including extrahepatic bile duct cancer) and pituitary tumors, Contraception 43:667, 1991.

113. Janerich DT, Dugan JM, Standfast SJ, Strite L, Congenital heart disease and prenatal exposure to exogenous sex hormones, Br Med J 1:1058, 1977.

114. Nora JJ, Nora AH, Blu J, Ingram J, Foster D, Exogenous progestogen and estrogen implicated in birth defects, JAMA 240:837, 1978.

115. Heinonen OP, Slone D, Monson RR, Hook EB, Shapiro S, Cardiovascular birth defects in antenatal exposure to female sex hormones, New Engl J Med 296:67, 1976.

116. Simpson JL, Phillips OP, Spermicides, hormonal contraception and congenital malformations, Adv Contracept 6:141, 1990.

117. Savolainen E, Saksela E, Saxen L, Teratogenic hazards of oral contraceptives analyzed in a national malformation register, Am J Obstet Gynecol 140:521, 1981.

118. Michaelis J, Michaelis H, Gluck E, Koller S, Prospective study of suspected associations between certain drugs administered during early pregnancy and congenital malformations, Teratology 27:57, 1983.

119. Bracken MB, Oral contraception and congenital malformations in offspring: A review and meta-analysis of the prospective studies, Obstet Gynecol 76:552, 1990.

120. Ressequie LJ, Hick JF, Bruen JA, et al, Congenital malformations among offspring exposed in utero to progestins, Olsted County, Minnesota, 1936–1974, Fertil Steril 43:514, 1985.

121. Katz Z, Lancet M, Skornik J, Chemke J, Mogilemer B, Klinberg M, Teratogenicity of progestogens given during the first trimester of pregnancy, Obstet Gynecol 65:775, 1985.

122. Vessey MP, Wright NH, McPherson K, Wiggins P, Fertility after stoping different methods of contraception, Br Med J 1:265, 1978.

123. Vessey MP, Smith MA, Yates D, Return of fertility after discontinuation of oral contraceptives: Influence of age and parity, Br J Fam Plann 11:120, 1986.

124. Linn S, Schoenbaum SC, Monson RR, Rosner B, Ryan KJ, Delay in conception for former 'pill' users, JAMA 247:629, 1982.

125. Bracken MB, Hellenbrand KG, Holford TR, Conception delay after oral contraceptive use: The effect of estrogen dose, Fertil Steril 53:21, 1990.

126. Rothman KJ, Fetal loss, twinning, and birth weight after oral-contraceptive use, New Engl J Med 297:468, 1977.

127. Rothman KJ, Liess J, Gender of offspring after oral-contraceptive use, New Engl J Med 295:859, 1976.

128. Magidor S, Poalti H, Harlap S, Baras M, Long-term follow-up of children whose mothers used oral contraceptives prior to contraception, Contraception 29:203, 1984.

129. Vessey M, Doll R, Peto R, Johnson B, Wiggins P, A long-term follow-up study of women using different methods of contraception—an interim report, J Biosoc Sci 8:373, 1976.

130. Royal College of General Practitioners, The outcome of pregnancy in former oral contraceptive users, Br J Obstet Gynaecol 83:608, 1976.

131. Betrabet SS, Shikary ZK, Toddywalla VS, Toddywalla SP, Patel D, Saxena BN, Transfer of norethisterone (NET) and levonorgestrel (LNG) from a single tablet into the infant's circulation through the mother's milk, Contraception 35:517, 1987.

132. Diaz S, Peralta O, Juez G, Herreros C, Casado ME, Salvatierra AM, Miranda P, Durn E, Croxatto HB, Fertility regulation in nursing women: III. Short-term influence of a low-dose combined oral contraceptive upon lactation and infant growth, Contraception 27:1, 1982.

133. Croxatto HB, Diaz S, Peralta O, Juez G, Herreros C, Casado ME, Salvatierra AM, Miranda P, Durn E, Fertility regulation in nursing women: IV. Long-term influence of a low-dose combined oral contraceptive initiated at day 30 postpartum upon lactation and child growth, Contraception 27:13, 1983.

134. Peralta O, Diaz S, Juez G, Herreros C, Casado ME, Salvatierra AM, Miranda P, Durn E, Croxatto HB, Fertility regulation in nursing women: V. Long-term influence of a low-dose combined oral contraceptive initiated at day 90 postpartum upon lactation and infant growth, Contraception 27:27, 1983.

135. WHO Task Force on Oral Contraceptives, Effects of hormonal contraceptives on milk volume and infant growth, Contraception 30:505, 1984.

136. Nilsson S, Mellbin T, Hofvander Y, Sundelin C, Valentin J, Nygren KG, Long-term follow-up of children breast-fed by mothers using oral contraceptives, Contraception 34:443, 1986.

137. Howie PW, McNeilly AS, Houston MJ, et al, Effect of supplementary food on suckling patterns and ovarian activity during lactation, Br Med J 282:757, 1981.

138. Perez A, Vela P, Masnick GS, Potter RG, First ovulation after childbirth: The effect of breastfeeding, Am J Obstet Gynecol 114:1041, 1972.

139. Diaz S, Peralta O, Juez G, Salvatierra AM, Casado ME, Duran E, Croxatto HB, Fertility regulation in nursing women. I. The probablity of conception in full nursing women living in an urban setting, J Biosoc Sci 14:329, 1982.

140. McNeilly AS, Glasier A, Howie PW, Endocrine control of lactational infertility, in Dobbing J, editor, *Maternal Nutrition and Lactational Infertility,* Nevey/Raven Press, New York, 1985, p. 177.

141. Rivera R, Kennedy KI, Ortiz E, Barrera M, Bhiwandiwala PP, Breast-feeding and the return to ovulation in Durango, Mexico, Fertil Steril 49:780, 1988.

142. Gray RH, Campbell OM, Apelo R, Eslami SS, Zacur H, Ramos RM, Gehret JC, Labbok MH, Risk of ovulation during lactation, Lancet 335:25, 1990.

143. Diaz S, Aravena R, Cardenas H, Casado ME, Miranda P, Schiappacasse V, Croxatto HB, Contraceptive efficacy of lactational amenorrhea in urban Chilean women, Contraception 43:335, 1991.

144. Pituitary Adenoma Study Group, Pituitary adenomas and oral contraceptives: A multicenter case-control study, Fertil Steril 39:753, 1983.

145. Shy FKK, McTiernan AM, Daling JR, Weiss NS, Oral contraceptive use and the occurrence of pituitary prolactinomas, JAMA 249:2204, 1983.

146. Wingrave SJ, Kay CR, Vessey MP, Oral contraceptives and pituitary adenomas, Br Med J 280:685, 1980.

147. Furuhjelm M, Carlstrom K, Amenorrhea following use of combined oral contraceptives, Acta Obstet Gynecol Scand 52:373. 1973.

148. Shearman RP, Smith ID, Statistical analysis of relationship between oral contraceptives, secondary amenorrhea and galactorrhea, J Obstet Gynecol Br Comwlth 79:654, 1972.

149. Jacobs HS, Knuth UA, Hull MGR, Franks S, Post "pill" amenorrhea—cause or coincidence? Br Med J 2:940, 1977.

150. Gray RH, Campbell OM, Zacur HA, Labbok MH, MacRae SL, Postpartum return of ovarian activity in nonbreastfeeding women monitored by urinary assays, J Clin Endocrinol Metab 64:645, 1987.

151. Washington AE, Cates W, Zaidi AA, Hospitalizations for pelvic inflammatory disease: Epidemiology and trends in the United States, 1975 to 1981, JAMA 251:2529, 1984.

152. Westrom I, Incidence, prevalence, and trends of acute pelvic inflammatory disease and its consequences in industrialized countries, Am J Obstet Gynecol 138:880, 1980.

153. Westrom L, Bengtsson LP, Mardh PA, The risk of pelvic inflammatory disease in women using intrauterine contraceptive devices as compared to non-users, Lancet ii:221, 1976.

154. Eschenbach DA, Harnisch JP, Holmes KK, Pathogenesis of acute pelvic inflammatory disease: Role of contraception and other risk factors, Am J Obstet Gynecol 128:838, 1977.

155. Rubin GL, Ory WH, Layde PM, Oral contraceptives and pelvic inflammatory disease, Am J Obstet Gynecol 140:630, 1980.

156. Senanayake P, Kramer DG, Contraception and the etiology of pelvic inflammatory diseases; New perspectives, Am J Obstet Gynecol 138:852, 1980.

157. Panser LA, Phipps WR, Type of oral contraceptive in relation to acute, initial episodes of pelvic inflammatory disease, Contraception 43:91, 1991.

158. Svensson L, Westrom L, Mardh P, Contraceptives and acute salpingitis, JAMA 251:2553, 1984.

159. Cates W Jr, Washington AE, Rubin GL, Peterson HB, The pill, chlamydia and PID, Fam Plann Persp 17:175, 1985.

160. Cramer DW, Goldman MB, Schiff I, Belisla S, Albrecht B, Stadel B, Gibson M, Wilson E, Stillman R, Thompson I, The relationship of tubal infertility to barrier method and oral contraceptive use, JAMA 257:2446, 1987.

161. Wolner-Hanssen P, Eschenbach DA, Paavonen J, Kiviat N, Stevens CE, Critchlow C, DeRouen T, Holmes KK, Decreased risk of symptomatic chlamydial pelvic inflammatory disease associated with oral contraceptive tuse, JAMA 263:54, 1990.

162. Hunter DJ, Mati JK, Contraception, family planning, and HIV, presented at the Conference on AIDS and Reproductive Health, Bellagio, Italy, 1990.

163. Barbone F, Austin H, Louv WC, Alexander WJ, A follow-up study of methods of contraception, sexual activity, and rates of trichomoniasis, candidiasis, and bacterial vaginosis, Am J Obstet Gynecol 163:510, 1990.

164. Ross RK, Pike MC, Vessey MP, Bull D, Yeates D, Casagrande JT, Risk factors for uterine fibroids: Reduced risk associated with oral contraceptives, Br Med J 293:359, 1986.

165. Mattson RH, Cramer JA, Darney PD, Naftolin F, Use of oral contraceptives by women with epilepsy, JAMA 256:238, 1986

166. Milsom I, Sundell G, Andersch B, A longitudinal study of contraception and pregnancy outcome in a representative sample of young Swedish women, Contraception 43:111, 1991.

167. Killick SR, Bancroft K, Oelbaum S, Morris J, Elstein M, Extending the duration of the pill-free interval during combined oral contraception, Adv Contraception 6:33, 1990.

168. Jung-Hoffman C, Kuhl H, Intra- and interindividual variations in contraceptive steroid levels during 12 treatment cycles: No relation to irregular bleedings, Contraception 42:423, 1990.

169. Grimes DA, Hughes JM, Use of multiphasic oral contraceptives and hospitalizations of women with functional ovarian cysts in the United States, Obstet Gynecol 73:1037, 1989.

170. Vessey M, Metcalfe A, Wells C, McPherson K, Westhoff C, Yeates D, Ovarian neoplasms, functional ovarian cysts, and oral contraceptives, Br Med J 294:1518, 1987.

171. Neely JL, Abate M, Swinker M, D'Angio R, The effect of doxycycline on serum levels of ethinyl estradiol, norethindrone, and endogenous progesterone, Obstet Gynecol 77:416, 1991.

172. Murphy AA, Zacur HA, Charache P, Burkman RT, The effect of tetracycline on levels of oral contraceptives, Am J Obstet Gynecol 164:28, 1991.

173. Szoka PR, Edgren RA, Drug interactions with oral contraceptives: Compilation and analysis of an adverse experience report database, Fertil Steril 49(Suppl):31S, 1988.

174. Abernethy DR, Greenblatt DJ, Divoll M, et al, Impairment of diazepam metabolism by low-dose estrogen-containing oral-contraceptive steroids, New Engl J Med 306:791, 1982.

175. Baciewicz AM, Oral contraceptive drug interactions, Ther Drug Monit 7:26, 1985.

176. Tornatore KM, Kanarkowski R, McCarthy TL, et al, Effect of chronic oral contraceptive steroids on theophylline disposition, Eur J Clin Pharmacol 23:129, 1982.

177. Mitchell MC, Hanew T, Meredith CG, et al, Effects of oral contraceptive steroids on acetaminophen metabolism and elimination, Clin Pharmacol Ther 34:48, 1983.

178. Gupta KC, Joshi JV, Hazari K, et al, Effect of low estrogen combination oral contraceptives on metabolism of aspirin and phenylbutazone, Int J Clin Pharmacol Ther Toxicol 20:511, 1982.

179. Jungers P, Dougados M, Pelissier L, et al, Influence of oral contraceptive therapy on the activity of systemic lupus erythematosus, Arthritis Rheum 25:618, 1982.

180. Lashner BA, Kane SV, Hanauer SB, Lack of association between OC use and ulcerative colitis, Gastroenterology 99:1032, 1990.

181. Coutinho EM, da Silva AR, Carreira C, Rodrigues V, Goncalves MT, Conception control by vaginal administration of pills containing ethinyl estradiol and dl-norgestrel, Fertil Steril 42:478, 1984.

182. Sullivan-Nelson M, Kuller JA, Zacur HA, Clinical use of oral contraceptives administered vaginally: A case report, Fertil Steril 52:864, 1989.

183. Milsom E, Sundell G, Andersch B, The influence of different combined oral contraceptives on the prevalence and severity of dysmenorrhea, Contraception 42:497, 1990.

184. Kirshon B, Poindexter AN III, Contraception: A risk factor for endometriosis, Obstet Gynecol 71:829, 1988.

185. Lindsay R, Tohme J, Kanders B, The effect of oral contraceptive use on vertebral bone mass in pre- and post-menopausal women, Contraception 34:333, 1986.

186. Lloyd T, Buchanan JR, Ursino GR, Myers C, Woodward G, Halbert DR, Long-term oral contraceptive use does not affect trabecular bone density, Am J Obstet Gynecol 160:402, 1989.

187. Enzelsberger H, Metka M, Heytmanek G, Schurz B, Kurz Ch, Kusztrich M, Influence of oral contraceptive use on bone density in climacteric women, Maturitas 9:375, 1988.

188. Kleerekoper M, Brienza RS, Schultz LR, Johnson CC, Oral contraceptive use may protect against low bone mass, Arch Intern Med 151:1971, 1991.

189. Spector TD, Roman E, Silman AJ, The pill, parity, and rheumatoid arthritis, Arthritis Rheum 33:782, 1990.

190. del Junco DJ, Annegers JF, Luthra HS, Coulam CB, Kurland LT, Do oral contraceptives prevent rheumatoid arthrits?, JAMA 254:1938, 1985.

191. Hazes JMW, Dijkmans BAC, Vandenbroucke JP, De Vries RRP, Cats A, Reduction of the risk of rheumatoid arthritis among women who take oral contraceptives, Arthritis Rheum 33:173, 1990.

192. Spector TD, Hochberg MC, The protective effect of the oral contraceptive pill on rheumatoid arthritis: An overview of the analytical epidemiological studies using meta-analysis, J Clin Epidemiol 43:1221, 1990.

193. van der Vange N, Blankenstein MA, Kloosterboer HJ, Haspels AA, Thijssen JHH, Effects of seven low-dose combined oral contraceptives on sex hormone binding globulin, corticosteroid binding globulin, total and free testsosterone, Contraception 41:345, 1990.

194. Lemay A, Dewailly SD, Grenier R, Huard J, Attenuation of mild hyperandrogenic activity in postpubertal acne by a triphasic oral contraceptive containing low doses of ethynyl estradiol and d,l-norgestrel, J Clin Endocrinol Metab 71:8, 1990.

195. Steinkampf MP, Hammond KR, Blackwell RE, Hormonal treatment of functional ovarian cysts: A randomized, prospective study, Fertil Steril 54:775, 1990.

196. Jones EF, Forrest JD, Contraceptive failure in the United States: Revised estimates from the 1982 National Survey of Family Growth, Fam Plann Perspect 21:103, 1989.

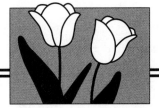

3

Special Uses of Oral Contraception:
The Progestin-Only Minipill
Emergency Contraception

ORAL CONTRACEPTION is a phrase which appropriately denotes a vast body of knowledge (Chapter 2)
pertaining to the combined estrogen-progestin "birth
control pill." However, there are two special types of oral contraception which deserve separate consideration, the progestin-only minipill
and emergency contraception.

The Progestin-Only Minipill

The minipill contains a small dose of a progestational agent and must
be taken daily, in a continuous fashion.[1,2] There is no evidence for any
difference in clinical behavior with any of the products.

Minipills available worldwide:

    1. Micronor, NOR-QD, Noriday, Norod ----0.350 mg
                     norethindrone
    2. Microval, Noregeston, Microlut ------------0.030 mg
                     levonorgestrel
    3. Ovrette, Neogest -----------------------------0.075 mg
                     norgestrel
    4. Exluton ---0.500 mg
                     lynestrenol
    5. Femulen --0.500 mg
                     ethynodial diacetate

Mechanism of Action

The small amount of progestin in the circulation will have a significant impact only on those tissues very sensitive to the female sex steroids, estrogen and progesterone. The contraceptive effect is more dependent upon endometrial and cervical mucus effects, since gonadotropins are not consistently suppressed. The endometrium involutes and becomes hostile to implantation, and the cervical mucus becomes thick and impermeable. Approximately 40% of patients will ovulate normally. Tubal physiology may also be affected, but this is speculative.

Because of the low dose, the minipill must be taken daily at the same time of day. The change in the cervical mucus requires 2–4 hours to take effect, and most importantly, the impermeability diminishes 22 hours after administration.

Ectopic pregnancy is not prevented as effectively as intrauterine pregnancy. Although the overall incidence of ectopic pregnancy is not increased, when pregnancy occurs, the clinician must suspect that it is more likely to be ectopic.

There are no significant metabolic effects[3], and there is an immediate return to fertility upon discontinuation (unlike the delay seen with the combination oral contraceptive).

Efficacy

Failure rates have been documented to range from 1.1 to 9.6 per 100 women in the first year of use.[4] The failure rate is higher in younger women (3.1 per 100 woman-years) compared to women over age 40 (0.3 per 100 woman-years).[5] In motivated women, the failure rate is comparable to the actual use rate with combination oral contraception.[6,7]

Pill Taking

The minipill should be started on the first day of menses, and a back-up method must be used for the first 7 days. The pill should be keyed to a daily event to ensure regular administration at the same time of the day. If pills are forgotten or gastrointestinal illness impairs absorption, the minipill should be resumed as soon as possible, and a back-up method should be used immediately and until the pills have been resumed for at least 2 days. If 2 or more pills are missed in a row and there is no menstrual bleeding in 4–6 weeks, a pregnancy test should be obtained. *If more than 3 hours late in taking a pill, a back-up method should be used for 48 hours.*

Problems

In view of the unpredictable effect on ovulation, it is not surprising that irregular menstrual bleeding is the major clinical problem. The daily progestational impact on the endometrium also contributes to this problem. Patients can expect to have normal, ovulatory cycles (40%), short, irregular cycles (40%), or a total lack of cycles ranging from irregular bleeding to spotting and amenorrhea (20%). This is the major reason why women discontinue the minipill method of contraception.[6]

Women on progestin-only contraception develop more functional, ovarian follicular cysts.[8] Nearly all, if not all, regress. This is not a clinical problem of any significance.

The levonorgestrel minipill may be associated with acne. The mechanism is similar to that seen with Norplant. The androgenic activity of levonorgestrel decreases the circulating levels of sex hormone binding globulin (SHBG). Therefore free steroid levels (levonorgestrel and testosterone) will be increased. This is in contrast to the action of combined oral contraception where the effect of the progestin is countered by the estrogen-induced increase in SHBG.

The incidence of the minor side effects is very low, probably at the same rate which would be encountered with a placebo.

Clinical Decisions

There are two situations where excellent efficacy, probably near total effectiveness, is achieved: lactating women and women over age 40. In lactating women, the contribution of the minipill is combined with prolactin-induced suppression of ovulation, adding up to very effective protection. In women over age 40, reduced fecundity adds to the minipill's effects.

There is another reason why the minipill is a good choice for the breastfeeding woman. There is no evidence for any adverse effect on breastfeeding as measured by milk volume and infant growth.[9] In fact, there is a modest positive impact; women using the minipill breastfeed longer and add supplementary feeding at a later time.[10] Because of the slight positive impact on lactation, the minipill can be started immediately after delivery.

The minipill is a good choice in situations where estrogen is contraindicated, such as patients with serious medical conditions (diabetes with vascular disease, severe systemic lupus erythematosus, cardiovascular disease). It should be noted that the freedom from estrogen effects, although likely, is presumptive. Substantial data, for example on associations with vascular disease, blood pressure, and cancer, are not available because relatively small numbers have chosen to use this method of contraception. On the other hand, it is very logical to conclude that any of the progestin effects associated with the combination oral contraceptives can be related to the minipill according to a dose-response curve; all effects should be reduced.

No impact can be measured on the coagulation system.[11] The minipill can probably be used in women with previous episodes of thrombosis, but the package insert in the United States carries the same precautions and warnings that combined oral contraceptives carry. This is not appropriate in view of the absence of estrogen and the lower dose of progestin. Theoretically, minipills should be free of serious complications. Unfortunately, the package insert injects an element of medical-legal risk for the clinician.

The minipill is a good alternative for the occasional woman who reports diminished libido on combination oral contraceptives, presumably due to decreased androgen levels. The minipill should also be considered for the few patients who report minor side effects (gastrointestinal upset, breast tenderness, headaches) of such a degree that the combination oral contraceptive is not acceptable.

Do the noncontraceptive benefits associated with combination oral contraception apply to the minipill? Studies are unable to help us with this issue, again because of relatively small numbers of users. However, the progestin impact on cervical mucus, endometrium, and ovulation leads one to think the benefits will be present, but probably at a reduced level.

Good efficacy with the minipill requires regularity, taking the pill at the same time each day. There is less room for forgetting, and therefore, the minipill is probably not a good choice for the noncompulsive, disorganized woman; and not a good choice for the average adolescent.

Emergency Contraception

The use of large doses of estrogen to prevent implantation was pioneered by Morris and van Wagenen at Yale in the 1960s. The initial work in monkeys led to the use of high doses of diethylstilbestrol (25–50 mg/day) and ethinyl estradiol in women.[12] It was quickly appreciated that these extremely large doses of estrogen were associated with a high rate of gastrointestinal side effects. Yuzpe developed a method utilizing a combination oral contraceptive, resulting in an important reduction in dosage.[13] The following treatment regimens have been documented to be effective:

> Conjugated Estrogen, 15 mg bid for 5 days, or 50 mg iv on each of 2 consecutive days.
> Ethinyl Estradiol, 2.5 mg bid for 5 days.
> Ovral, 4 tablets (2 given 12 hours apart).

This method has been more commonly called postcoital contraception, or the "morning after" treatment. Emergency contraception is a more accurate and appropriate name, indicating the intention to be one-time protection. It is an important option for patients, and should be considered when condoms break, sexual assault occurs, if diaphragms or cervical caps dislodge, or with the lapsed use of any method. In a study at an abortion service, fully half of the patients would have been suitable for emergency contraception.[14] Emergency contraception is another component of contraception that cries for public education and media publicity.

Mechanism and Efficacy

The mechanism of action is not known with certainty, but it is believed with justification that this treatment interferes with implantation. The efficacy has been confirmed in large clinical trials and summarized in a complete review of the literature.[15] Treatment with high doses of estrogen yields a failure rate of approximately 1%, with the combination oral contraceptive, about 2%. The failure rate is lowest with high doses of ethinyl estradiol given within 72 hours (0.1%), but the side effects make the combination oral contraceptive a better choice.

Treatment Method

Treatment should be initiated as soon after exposure as possible, but no later than 72 hours. Because of possible, but unlikely, harmful effects of these high doses to a fetus, an already existing pregnancy should be ruled out prior to use of postcoital hormones. Furthermore, the patient should be offered therapeutic abortion if the method fails. This patient encounter also provides an important opportunity to screen for STDs.

The combination oral contraceptive method delivers significantly less steroid hormone, and this reduction in the total dose and the number of doses reduces the side effects and limits them to a shorter time period. It is worth adding an antiemetic, oral or suppository, to the treatment. Side effects reflect the high doses used: nausea, vomiting, breast tenderness, headache, and dizziness. The usual contraindications for oral contraception apply to this use.

A 3 week follow-up visit should be scheduled to assess the result, and to counsel for regular contraception.

Could other combination oral contraceptive products be used? Since other doses and other formulations have never been tested, the efficacy is unknown. It would not be appropriate to expose patients to an unknown failure rate.

Another method of emergency contraception is the insertion of a copper IUD, up to 5 days after unprotected intercourse. The failure rate (in a small number of studies) is very low, 0.1%.[15] This method definitely prevents implantation, but it is not suitable for nulliparous women or women at risk for infection (multiple sexual partners, rape victim).

References

1. Fotherby K, The progestogen-only pill, Br J Fam Plann 8:7, 1982.

2. Graham S, Fraser IS, The progestogen-only mini-pill, Contraception 26:373, 1982.

3. Ball MJ, Gillmer AE, Progestagen-only oral contraceptives: Comparison of the metabolic effects of levonorgestrel and norethisterone, Contraception 44:223, 1991.

4. Trussell J, Kost K, Contraceptive failure in the United States: A critical review of the literature, Stud Fam Plann 18:237, 1987.

5. Vessey MP, Lawless M, Yeates D, McPherson K, Progestogen-only contraception: Findings in a large prospective study with special reference to effectiveness, Br J Fam Plann 10:117, 1985.

6. Broome M, Fotherby K, Clinical experience with the progestogen-only pill, Contraception 42:489, 1990.

7. Seth A, Jain U, Sharma S, et al, A randomized, double-blind study of two combined and two progestogen-only oral contraceptives, Contraception 25:243, 1982.

8. Tayob Y, Adams J, Jacobs HS, Guillebaud J, Ultrasound demonstration of increased frequency of functional ovarian cysts in women using progestogen-only oral contraception, Br J Obstet Gynaecol 92:1003, 1985.

9. WHO Special Programme of Research, Development, and Research Training in Human Reproduction, Task Force on Oral Contraceptives, Effects of hormonal contraceptives on milk volume and infant growth, Contraception 30:505, 1984.

10. McCann MF, Moggia AV, Hibbins JE, Potts M, Becker C, The effects of a progestin-only oral contraceptive (levonorgestrel 0.03 mg) on breast-feeding, Contraception 40:635, 1989.

11. Fotherby K, The progestogen-only pill and thrombosis, Br J Fam Plann 15:83, 1989.

116

12. Morris J McL, van Wagenen G, Compounds interfering with ovum implantation and development. III. The role of estrogens, Am J Obstet Gynecol 96:804, 1966.

13. Yuzpe AA, Smith RP, Rademaker AW, A multicenter clinical investigation employing ethinyl estradiol combined with dl-norgestrel as a postcoital contraceptive agent, Fertil Steril 37:508, 1982.

14. Burton R, Savage W, Reader F, The "morning after pill." Is this the wrong name for it? Br J Fam Plann 15:119, 1990.

15. Fasoli M, Parazzini F, Cecchetti G, La Vecchia C, Post-coital contraception: An overview of published studies, Contraception 39:459, 1989.

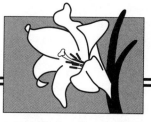

4

Long-Acting Steroid Methods

THE SUSTAINED-RELEASE systems for delivering progestins are the first clinical innovation available in contraception since oral contraception was introduced and IUDs were
re-discovered in the 1960s.[1] The first of these new methods, Norplant,
employs silastic tubing permeable to steroid molecules to provide
stable circulating levels of synthetic progestins over months and
years. The progestins, circulating at levels one-fourth to one-tenth of
those obtained with combined oral contraceptives, prevent conception by suppressing ovulation and thickening cervical mucus to
inhibit sperm penetration so that fertilization rarely occurs.[2]

Injectable medroxyprogesterone acetate (Depo-Provera) is a long-
acting (3–6 months) agent which has been part of the contraceptive
programs of many countries for more than 20 years. This experience
has demonstrated it to be safe, effective, and acceptable. It is not a
"sustained release" system, but its action is the same.

Because serum levels of progestin remain low and because no estrogen
is administered, these long-acting contraceptive methods have not
caused any serious health effects.[3] These methods do, however, cause
many of the same minor, but bothersome, side effects associated with
the progestin component of combined oral contraceptives. The
continuous presence of low levels of progestin leads to irregular
endometrial sloughing, a problem common to all of these methods,
and one which is highly variable from one woman to another.

The efficacy of long-acting progestin systems compares favorably to sterilization, oral contraception, and IUDs.[4] An important contribution to efficacy in actual use is the nature of the delivery systems themselves which require little effort on the part of the user. Since compliance does not require frequent resupply or instruction in use, as with oral contraception, theoretical (lowest expected) effectiveness is very close to the actual or typical (use) effectiveness.

Sustained-release methods require less of the user but they demand more of the clinician. Norplant involves minor operative procedures for placement and for discontinuation. Disturbances of menstrual patterns and other side effects prompt many more questions from patients about these new methods than about use of the familiar oral, intrauterine, and barrier contraceptives. In addition, clinicians have a special responsibility to become skillful in the minor operations required to remove implants and to be available to women when those skills are required to terminate use.

Because Norplant is available for use in the U.S., our attention will be directed to this particular method. Our descriptions are intended to provide a foundation for learning the techniques unique for the use of Norplant, but not to serve as a substitute for clinical instruction. Skill in insertion and removal operations are best acquired from someone already experienced in these procedures.

The Norplant System

The Norplant subdermal implant system is a long-acting, low-dose, reversible, progestin-only method of contraception for women. It was developed by the Population Council. The implants are manufactured, under license of the Population Council, by Huhtamaki Oy/Leiras Pharmaceuticals in Finland.

Norplant was first introduced into clinical trials in Chile in 1972.[5] Assessment of this method has been completed in more than 45 countries.[3] In 1990, Norplant was approved for marketing in the U.S., the twentieth country to do so.

Description

The Norplant system consists of 6 capsules, each measuring 34 mm in length with a 2.4 mm outer diameter and containing levonorgestrel. The capsule is made of flexible, medical grade Silastic (polydimethylsiloxane) tubing which is sealed shut with Silastic medical adhesive, silicone type A. The cavity of the capsule has an inner diameter of 1.57 mm, with an inner length of 30 mm. Each capsule contains 36 mg of dry crystalline levonorgestrel for a total of 216 mg in the 6 capsules. The levonorgestrel is very stable and has remained unchanged in capsules examined after more than 7 years of use.

The implants come packaged in heat-sealed pouches that have a shelf life of 5 years from the date of manufacture and have an additional 5 year effective life once inserted. Storage at room temperature with uncontrolled humidity has not altered their composition or lifespan after 4 years, but optimally the implants should be stored in a cool, dry area away from direct sunlight. The implants can be ethylene oxide sterilized, but cannot be sterilized by ionizing radiation, dry heat, or autoclaving.

The components of Norplant are not new. The silastic in the tubing has been used in surgical applications such as prosthetic devices, heart valves, and drainage tubes, since the 1950s. The progestin, levonorgestrel, has been widely used in oral contraceptives since the 1960s. The toxicology, teratogenicity, and pharmacology of levonorgestrel have been well studied. What is new is the way the system delivers a sustained level of levonorgestrel for a long time.

Release Rates. The release rate of the capsule is determined by its total surface area and the thickness of the capsule wall. The levonorgestrel diffuses through the wall of the tubing into the surrounding tissues where it is absorbed by the circulatory system and distributed systemically, avoiding an initial high level in the hepatic circulation. Within 24 hours after insertion, plasma concentrations of levonorgestrel range from 0.4 to 0.5 ng/ml, high enough to prevent conception.[6]

The capsules release approximately 80 µg of levonorgestrel per 24 hours during the first 6–12 months of use. This rate declines gradually to 30–35 µg per day for the remaining duration of use. After 5 years, the implants release about 25 µg per day. The 80 µg per day of hormone released by the implants during the first 2–6 months of use is about the same as the daily dose of levonorgestrel delivered by the progestin-only, minipill oral contraceptive, and 25–50% of the dose delivered by low dose combined oral contraceptives.

Mean plasma concentrations below 0.20 ng/ml are associated with increased pregnancy rates. After 6 months of use, daily levonorgestrel concentrations are about 0.35 ng/ml; at 2.5 years, the levels decrease to 0.25–0.35 ng/ml. Until the 5 year mark, mean levels remain above 0.25 ng/ml.[7]

Body weight affects the circulating levels of levonorgestrel. The greater the weight of the user, the lower the levonorgestrel concentrations at any time during Norplant use. The greatest decrease over time occurs in women weighing more than 70 kg (154 pounds).

Levonorgestrel levels may also be affected by the levels of sex hormone binding globulin (SHBG). Levonorgestrel has a high affinity for SHBG. In the week after Norplant insertion, SHBG levels decline rapidly, then return to about half of preinsertion levels by 1 year of use. This effect on SHBG is not uniform and may account for some of the individual variations in plasma levonorgestrel concentrations.[8]

Mechanism of Action

The mechanism by which Norplant prevents conception is only partially explained. There are three probable modes of action, which are similar to those attributed to the contraceptive effect of the progestin-only, minipills:

1. The levonorgestrel suppresses at both the hypothalamus and the pituitary the luteinizing hormone (LH) surge necessary for ovulation. As determined by progesterone levels in many users over several years, about one-third of all cycles are ovulatory.[7,9]
2. The levonorgestrel has a marked effect on the cervical mucus. The mucus thickens and decreases in amount, forming a barrier to sperm penetration.[6,10]
3. The constant level of levonorgestrel suppresses the estradiol-induced cyclic maturation of the endometrium, and eventually causes atrophy. These changes could prevent implantation should fertilization occur, however no evidence of fertilization can be detected in Norplant users.[11]

Advantages

Norplant is a safe, highly effective, continuous method of contraception which requires little user compliance or motivation and is rapidly reversible. Because this is a progestin-only method, it may be utilized by women who have contraindications for the use of estrogen-containing oral contraceptives. The sustained release of low doses of progestin avoids the high initial dose delivered by injectables and the daily hormone surge associated with oral contraceptives. Norplant is not a coitus-related contraceptive method. The use-effectiveness closely approximates the theoretical effectiveness.

Disadvantages

There are some disadvantages associated with the use of the Norplant system:

1. Norplant frequently causes disruption of bleeding patterns in up to 80% of users, especially during the first year of use, and some women or their partners find these changes unacceptable.[12] Endogenous estrogen is variably suppressed, and unlike the combined oral contraceptives, no exogenous estrogen is provided to maintain a stable endometrium. The absence of cyclic administration does not allow for regular withdrawal bleeding. Consequently, the relatively unstable endometrium sheds at unpredictable intervals.

2. The implants must be inserted and removed in a surgical procedure performed by trained personnel. Women cannot initiate or discontinue the method without the assistance of a clinician.

3. Because the insertion and removal of Norplant requires a minor surgical procedure, initiation and discontinuation costs will be higher than with oral contraceptives or barrier methods.

4. The implants can be visible under the skin. This sign of the use of contraception may be unacceptable for some women, and for some partners.[12]

5. Norplant is not known to provide protection against sexually transmitted diseases (STDs) such as herpes, human papillomavirus, HIV, gonorrhea, or chlamydia. Users at risk for STDS must consider adding a barrier method to prevent infection.

Indications

The Norplant system is indicated for use by women of reproductive age who are sexually active and desire continuous contraception. Norplant should be considered for women who:

1. Desire spacing of future pregnancies.
2. Desire a highly effective, long-term method of contraception.
3. Experience serious or minor estrogen-related side effects with oral contraception.
4. Have difficulty remembering to take pills every day, have contraindications or difficulty using IUDs, or desire a non-coitus-related method of contraception.
5. Have completed their childbearing but do not desire permanent sterilization.
6. Have a history of anemia with heavy menstrual bleeding.
7. Are considering sterilization, but are not yet ready to undergo surgery.
8. Have chronic illnesses and whose health will be threatened by pregnancy.

Absolute Contraindications

Norplant use is contraindicated in women who have:

1. *ACTIVE* thrombophlebitis or thromboembolic disease.
2. Undiagnosed genital bleeding.
3. *ACUTE* liver disease.
4. Benign or malignant liver tumors.
5. Known or suspected breast cancer.

Relative Contraindications

Based on clinical judgment and appropriate medical management, Norplant *MAY BE USED* by women with a history of or current diagnosis of the following conditions:

1. Heavy cigarette smoking (15 or more daily) in women older than 35 years.
2. History of ectopic pregnancy.

3. Diabetes mellitus. Because multiple studies have failed to observe a significant impact on carbohydrate metabolism, Norplant, in our view, is particularly well-suited for diabetic women.
4. Hypercholesterolemia.
5. Severe acne.
6. Hypertension.
7. History of cardiovascular disease, including myocardial infarction, cerebral vascular accident, coronary artery disease, or angina. Patients with artificial heart valves.
8. Gallbladder disease.
9. Severe vascular or migraine headaches.
10. Severe depression.
11. Chronic disease, such as immunocompromized patients.
12. Concomitant use of medications that induce microsomal liver enzymes (phenytoin, phenobarbital, carbamazepine, rifampin). In this case, we do not recommend the use of Norplant because of a likely increased risk of pregnancy due to lower blood levels of levonorgestrel.

Efficacy

Norplant is a more effective method of birth control than any of the other reversible methods. In studies conducted in 11 countries, totaling 12,133 woman-years of use, the pregnancy rate was 0.2 pregnancies per 100 woman-years of use.[3] All but one of the pregnancies that occurred during this evaluation were present at the time of implant insertion. If these luteal phase insertions are excluded from analysis, the first year pregnancy rate was 0.01 per 100 woman-years.

Failure Rates During the First Year of Use, United States [4]

Method	Percent of Women with Pregnancy Lowest Expected	Typical
No method	85.0%	85.0%
Combination Pill	0.1	3.0
Progestin only	0.5	3.0
IUDs		3.0
Progesterone IUD	2.0	<2.0
Copper T 380A	0.8	<1.0
Norplant	0.2	0.2
Female sterilization	0.2	0.4
Male sterilization	0.1	0.15
Depo-Provera	0.3	0.3
Spermicides	3.0	21.0
Periodic abstinence		20.0
Calendar	9.0	
Ovulation method	3.0	
Symptothermal	2.0	
Post–ovulation	1.0	
Withdrawal	4.0	18.0
Cervical cap	6.0	18.0
Sponge		
Parous women	9.0	28.0
Nulliparous women	6.0	18.0
Diaphragm and spermicides	6.0	18.0
Condom	2.0	12.0

124

The overall pregnancy rate after 2 years of use in 9 countries was 0.2 per 100 woman-years of use.[3] The pregnancy rate achieved in the U.S. trials during the second year of use was higher (2.1 per 100 woman-years). Two factors may account for this difference. First, users in the U.S. weighed, on the average, more than study participants in other countries. Clinical trials have demonstrated a direct correlation between weight greater than 70 kg (154 pounds) and an increased risk of pregnancy, but even for heavy women, pregnancy rates are lower than with oral contraception. Second, two different types of Silastic tubing were used in the manufacture of Norplant capsules.[13] The first type contained a larger proportion of inert filler and was more dense, while the second type contained less filler and was less dense. Higher pregnancy rates have been observed among women using the more dense capsules, and in the U.S. trials, capsules were more often of the more dense variety. The less dense tubing is now the only one used in the manufacture of Norplant and has a 15% higher release rate than denser tubing.

Pregnancy Rates According to Years of Use [3]

First Year	Second Year	Third Year	Fourth Year	Fifth Year
0.2%	0.2%	0.9%	0.5%	1.1%

Using the less dense tubing, there now are no weight restrictions for Norplant users, but heavier women (more than 70 kg) may experience slightly higher pregnancy rates in the fourth and fifth years of use compared to lighter women. Even in the later years, however, pregnancy rates for heavier women using Norplant are lower than with oral contraception. The differences in pregnancy rates by weight are probably due to the dilutional effect of larger body size on the low, sustained serum levels of levonorgestrel. Heavier women should not rely on Norplant beyond the 5 year limit. For slender women the duration of Norplant's efficacy may extend well into the fifth year of use.

Norplant is less effective in women who are also using drugs which accelerate hepatic microsomal metabolism. These drugs include phenytoin (Dilantin), carbamazepine (Tegretrol), phenobarbitol, and rifampin. Since serum levels are already low, rapid metabolism can push them under the contraceptive level. For women with compromised hepatic function, the low serum levels of levonorgestrel present no metabolic problem because even if excretion is impaired, levels will not become very high.

Ectopic Pregnancy

The ectopic pregnancy rate during Norplant use has been 0.28 per 1,000 woman-years.[3] This compares to the rate of 1.5 per 1,000 among U.S. women aged 15–44.[14] *Although the risk of developing an ectopic pregnancy during use of Norplant is low, when pregnancy does occur, ectopic pregnancy should be suspected, especially if the patient has additional risk factors.*

Ectopic Pregnancy Rates per 1,000 Woman-Years [3, 14, 15]

All U.S. women	1.50
Non-contraceptive users	3.00
Copper T-380 IUD	0.20
Norplant	0.28

Menstrual Effects

Menstrual bleeding patterns are highly variable among users of Norplant. Some alteration of menstrual patterns will occur during the first year of use in approximately 60% of users.[16] The changes include alterations in the interval between bleeding, the duration and volume of menstrual flow, and spotting. Oligomenorrhea and amenorrhea also occur, but are less common. Irregular and prolonged bleeding usually occurs during the first year. Although bleeding problems occur much less frequently after the second year, they can occur at any time.[17]

Menstrual Patterns of Norplant Users [5, 6]

Menstrual Pattern	First Year	Second Year	Third Year
8 or more days bleeding	44%	27%	24%
15 or more days bleeding	15%	4%	7%
70 or more days without bleeding	37%	30%	22%
90 or more days without bleeding	26%	19%	15%
Bleeding days	54 days	48 days	48 days

Despite an increase in the number of spotting and bleeding days over preinsertion menstrual patterns, hemoglobin concentrations rise in Norplant users because of a decrease in the average amount of menstrual blood loss.[19]

Patients who can no longer tolerate the presence of prolonged bleeding will benefit from a short course of oral estrogen: conjugated estrogen, 1.25 mg, or estradiol, 2 mg, administered daily for 7 days. A therapeutic dose of one of the prostaglandin inhibitors given during the bleeding will help to diminish flow, but estrogen is more effective.[20]

Although, the Norplant system is very effective, pregnancy must be considered in women reporting amenorrhea who have been ovulating previously, as evidenced by regular menses prior to an episode of amenorrhea. A sensitive urine pregnancy test should be obtained. Women who remain amenorrheic throughout their use of Norplant are unlikely to become pregnant.[17] It is important to explain to patients the mechanism of the amenorrhea: the local progestational effect causing decidualization and atrophy.

Metabolic Effects

Exposure to the sustained, low dose of levonorgestrel delivered by the implants is not associated with significant metabolic changes. Studies of carbohydrate metabolism,[21,22] liver function,[23,24] blood coagulation,[25] immunoglobulin levels,[21,26] serum cortisol levels,[27] and blood chemistries[21,24,28] have failed to detect changes outside of normal ranges.

No major impact on the lipoprotein profile can be demonstrated.[2,28] Minor changes are transient, and with prolonged duration of use, lipoproteins return to preinsertion levels.[24,28] Long-term exposure to the low dose of levonorgestrel released by Norplant is unlikely to affect users' risk of atherosclerosis, just as prolonged exposure to combined oral contraception has not (see Chapter 2).

Effects on Future Fertility

Circulating levels of levonorgestrel become too low to measure within 48 hours after removal of Norplant. Most women resume normal ovulatory cycles during the first month after removal. The pregnancy rates during the first year after removal are comparable to those of women not using contraceptive methods and trying to become pregnant. There are no long-term effects on future fertility, nor are there any effects on sex ratios, rates of ectopic pregnancy, spontaneous abortion, stillbirth, or congenital malformations.[3]

Side Effects

The occurrence of serious side effects is very rare. In addition to the menstrual changes, the following side effects have been reported: headache, acne, weight change, mastalgia, hyperpigmentation over the implants, hirsutism, depression, mood changes, anxiety, nervousness, ovarian cyst formation, and galactorrhea.[3,12,16] It is difficult, of course, to be certain which of these effects were actually caused by the levonorgestrel. Although these side effects are minor in nature, they can cause patients to discontinue the method. Patients often find common side effects tolerable after assurance that they do not represent a health hazard.[12] Many complaints respond to reassurance; others can be treated with simple therapies. The most common side effect experienced by users is headache; about 20% of women who discontinue use do so because of headache.

Weight Change. Women using Norplant more frequently complain of weight gain than of weight loss, but findings are variable. In the Dominion Republic, 75% of those who changed weight lost, while in San Francisco, two-thirds gained. Assessment of weight change in Norplant users is confounded by changes in exercise, diet, and aging. Although an increase in appetite can be attributed to the androgenic activity of levonorgestrel, it is unlikely that the low levels with Norplant have any clinical impact. Counseling for weight changes should include dietary review and focus on dietary changes.

Mastalgia. Bilateral mastalgia, often occurring premenstrually, is usually associated with complaints of fluid retention. After pregnancy has been ruled out, reassurance and therapy aimed at symptomatic relief are indicated. This symptom decreases with increasing duration of Norplant use. Most Norplant users respond to treatment and do not elect to remove the implants. Careful assessments of the relationship between methylxanthines and mastalgia have failed to demonstrate a link. The most effective treatments are the following: danazol (200 mg/day), vitamin E (600 units/day), bromocriptine (2.5 mg/day), or tamoxifen (20 mg/day).

Galactorrhea. Galactorrhea is more common among women who have had insertion of the implants upon discontinuation of lactation. Pregnancy and other possible causes should be ruled out by performing a pregnancy test and a thorough breast examination. Patients should be reassured that this is a common occurrence among implant and oral contraceptive users. Decreasing the amount of breast and nipple stimulation during sexual relations can alleviate the symptom, but if amenorrhea accompanies persistent galactorrhea, a prolactin level should be obtained (see Chapter 12).

Acne. Acne, with or without an increase in oil production, is the most common skin complaint among Norplant users. The acne is caused by the androgenic activity of the levonorgestrel which produces a direct impact and also causes a decrease in sex hormone binding globulin (SHBG) levels leading to an increase in free steroid levels (both levonorgestrel and testosterone). This is in contrast to combined oral contraceptives which contain levonorgestrel, where the estrogen effect on SHBG (an increase) produces a decrease in unbound, free androgens. Common therapies for complaints of acne include dietary change, practice of good skin hygiene with the use of soaps or skin cleansers, and application of topical antibiotics (e.g. 1% clindamycin solution or gel, or topical erythromycin). Use of local antibiotics helps most users to continue Norplant.

Ovarian Cysts. Unlike oral contraception, the low serum progestin levels maintained by Norplant do not suppress FSH which continues to stimulate ovarian follicle growth in some users. The LH peak, on the other hand, is usually abolished so that these follicles do not ovulate. However, some continue to grow and cause pain or are palpated at the time of pelvic examination. Adnexal masses are approximately 8 times more frequent in Norplant users compared to normally cycling women. Because these are simple cysts (and most regress spontaneously within one month of detection), they need not be sonographically or laparoscopically evaluated. Further evaluation is indicated if they became large and painful or fail to regress. Regular ovulators are less likely to form cysts.

Herpes Simplex. Some users have complained of outbreaks of genital herpes simplex lesions occurring more frequently than prior to insertion. Most commonly, the lesions develop during periods of prolonged spotting or bleeding with the wearing of sanitary napkins. Use of vaginal tampons for bleeding and suppression of the virus with oral acyclovir (200 mg tid for up to 6 months) have been sucessful in dealing with this problem.

Patient Evaluation

The usual personal and family medical history and physical examination should concentrate on factors that might contraindicate use of the various contraceptive options. If a patient elects to use Norplant, a detailed description of the method, including effectiveness, side effects, risks, benefits, as well as insertion and removal procedures, should be provided. Before insertion, the patient should read and sign a written consent for the surgical placement of Norplant. It should include a review of the potential complications of the procedure which include reaction to the local anesthetic, infection, expulsion of the implants, superficial phlebitis, and bruising.

Insertion can be performed at any time during the menstrual cycle as long as pregnancy can be ruled out. If the patient's last menstrual period was abnormal, if she has recently had sexual intercourse without contraception, or if there are reasons to suspect pregnancy, a sensitive urine pregnancy test should be performed. Norplant can be inserted immediately postpartum, but certainly should be initiated no later than the third postpartum week.

Patients should be questioned regarding allergies to local anesthetics, antiseptic solutions, and tape. A discussion about the technique of insertion and anticipated sensations is an important part of preparing the patient for the experience. All patients approach insertion with some degree of apprehension which can be decreased by detailed explanations and preparation.[12]

Selection of the site for placement of Norplant is based on both functional and aesthetic factors. Various sites (the upper leg, forearm, and upper arm) have been used in clinical trials. The nondominant, upper, inner arm is usually the best site. This area is easily accessible to the clinician with minimal exposure of the patient. It is well protected during most normal activities. It is not highly visible, and it minimizes migration of the implants. The site of placement does not affect circulating levonorgestrel levels.

Insertion Technique

Insertion is carried out under local anesthesia in the office or clinic by someone, usually a physician or nurse practitioner, trained in the technique described here. The procedure takes 5–10 minutes.

Proper insertion is important for easy removal later. If the implants are placed just under and parallel to the skin (subdermally) with the tips near the insertion site close together and with their opposite ends far apart in a fan-shaped distribution, removal will be easier than if they are deeply placed and not fanned out.

Required Equipment.
- 6 cc syringe.
- 1.5 inch, 18-gauge needle for drawing up the anesthetic.
- 1.5 inch, 22-gauge needle for injecting the anesthetic.
- Sterile 4 x 4 gauze sponges.
- 1% chloroprocaine or lidocaine without epinephrine.
- Antiseptic solution.
- No. 11 scalpel.
- Steristrips or butterfly closures.
- Elastic bandage.
- A specially marked 10-gauge trocar with a blunt obturator.
- The 6 implants.
- Sterile gloves.
- 3 sterile drapes (under the arm, fenestrated over the arm, sterile field for supplies).

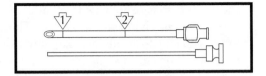

The specially marked trocar bears two marks along the length of the barrel to aid in the correct placement of the implants. The first mark is close to the bevel and indicates how far the trocar should be retracted before redirecting it for placement of subsequent implants. The second mark is close to the hub and indicates the length of the trocar that must be inserted under the skin prior to loading the implants for placement.

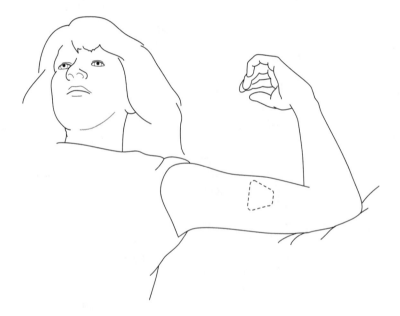

Positioning the Patient. The patient is placed in a supine position with the full length of her arm exposed. The upper inner arm is positioned by bending the elbow to 90° and rotating the arm out, allowing full exposure of the insertion site at the medial aspect of the bicep. Adequate support under the arm should be provided to ensure comfort. To minimize the risk of infection, strict aseptic technique should be maintained throughout the procedure. A sterile drape is placed under the arm, and a 10 x 10 cm area of skin on the upper arm is cleaned with an antiseptic such as povidone-iodine. An insertion site approximately 4 fingerbreadths (8–12 cm) superior and lateral to the medial epicondyle of the humerus is identified.

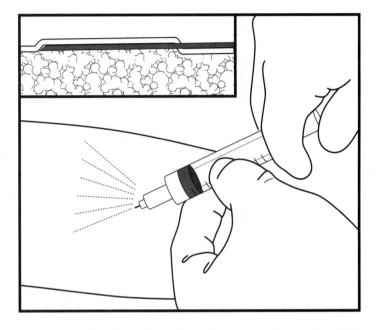

Anesthesia. Local anesthesia for the incision is obtained by raising a wheal of 1% chloroprocaine or lidocaine using a 22-gauge needle. the needle is then advanced under the skin its full length to its hub, and 1 ml of anesthetic is injected as it is withdrawn. The needle is advanced 5 more times to create, in the shape of a fan, an anesthetic field with 6 channels along which the implants will be placed. This requires about 6 ml of anesthetic. Injection of the anesthetic along these channels raises the dermis from the underlying tissue and allows easier introduction of the trocar.

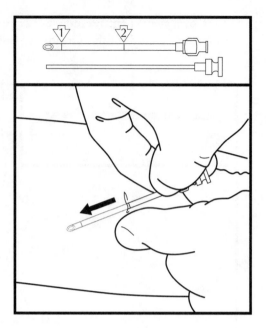

Incision and Placement. The no. 10 trocar and its obturator can usually be pushed directly through the skin without first making an incision, but if the skin is tough, a 2 mm skin incision is made with the no. 11 scalpel at the selected site 8–12 cm above the medial humeral epicondyle. The trocar with obturator in place is advanced as superficially as possible under the skin by maintaining an upward angle on the trocar. The trocar should elevate the skin at all times, and it should not be forced into the skin. If resistance is met, a slightly different angle to the left or right should be tried, along with a rotation of the trocar under the skin. If dimpling is seen, the trocar is not sufficiently underneath the skin.

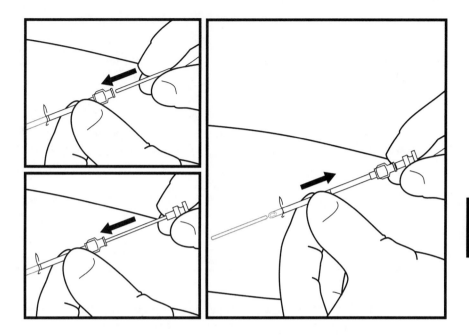

Once the trocar has been advanced to the mark nearest the hub (4.5 cm), the obturator is removed, and the first implant is loaded into the trocar. The obturator is replaced and used to advance the implant to the end of the trocar until slight, initial resistance is met. Holding the obturator stationary, the trocar is completely retracted over the obturator leaving the implant behind. Pushing on the obturator while withdrawing the trocar will advance the implant too far into the tissue, resulting in poor alignment with the distal tips of the other implants. After the trocar is completely retracted on the obturator, gentle downward pressure is exerted on the proximal end of the implant while retracting the trocar and obturator together to the mark closest to the bevel. This will ensure that the distal tip of the implant lies at least 0.5 cm above the incision.

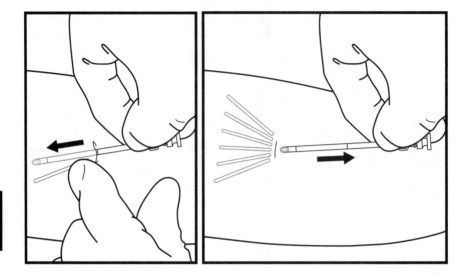

The trocar is not removed from the incision until all implants have been placed. With the obturator advanced fully into the trocar, the direction of the trocar is changed so that the next implant will lie at a 15 degree angle from the previous implant, forming a fanlike distribution of the 6 implants. A finger is placed on the previous implant and with gentle downward pressure, its position is fixed while advancing the trocar to the mark near the hub for placement of the next implant. Placement of a finger over the previous implant will ensure adequate spacing and prevent inadvertent puncture of the implant already placed. The obturator is removed, and the second implant is loaded and placed. The procedure is repeated for each implant to be inserted.

Most women experience little pain during the insertion. The most commonly reported discomfort is a burning sensation during the injection of the local anesthetic. This effect of local anesthetic can be eliminated for most patients by adding 1 meq of sodium bicarbonate to each 10 ml of anesthetic (this shortens shelf life to 24 hours). After the onset of anesthesia in 2–3 minutes, most women feel no more than a pressure sensation.

Closure. After all the implants have been inserted, the skin is closed with an adhesive strip. Sutures are not required. The insertion site is covered with two sterile 4 x 4 gauze sponges. An elastic bandage is wrapped around the upper arm to create a pressure dressing.

After completing the insertion, the placement of the implants should be documented with a drawing in the medical record, indicating the relationship of each implant to the others. The patient should be advised that there may be bruising around the implants. The pressure dressing should be kept in place for 24 hours (longer if an obvious hematoma develops during insertion), and the adhesive strip until it falls off (usually in 3–5 days). Pain is unusual, but if it occurs it can be relieved with aspirin, acetaminophen, or nonsteroidal anti-inflammatory agents. Infection or expulsion of the implants is rare (less than 1%), and usually occurs when an implant is left pressing against the wound. The clinician should be called for local pain, discharge, or swelling, or fever.

Complications of Insertion

Potential complications include infection, hematoma formation, local irritation or rash over the implants, expulsion of one or more of the implants, and allergic reactions to adhesives or the dressing. The incidence of complications is minimized by clinician training and experience, and the use of strict aseptic technique.

Infection. The rate of infection varies among clinics and countries. The overall risk of infection after Norplant insertion is 0.8%.[29] Infections usually occur within the first week after insertion, but can present as long as 4–5 months later. Infection can be treated either by the removal of the implants or the administration of oral antibiotics while the implants remain in place. One-third of insertion site infections treated with antibiotics are unresponsive to therapy and require removal.[29] There have been no reports of infections leading to serious injury. Rarely, a superficial phlebitis develops. If it resolves over 1–2 weeks with heat and elevation of the arm, the implants need not be removed.

Expulsion. Expulsion of one or more of the implants occurs in 0.4% of users, usually within the first few months of use.[29] The majority of expulsions are associated with concurrent infection at the insertion site. Another cause of expulsion is failure to advance the implants far enough from the incision, causing pressure on the incision by the distal tip of the implant. If an implant is expelled without evidence of infection, a new one can be inserted. If a new implant cannot be inserted within a few weeks, then the remaining implants should be removed. Remember to remind the patient that another method of contraception should be used while waiting for reinsertion.

Local Reactions. Although not common, hematomas can form when Norplant is inserted. The use of a pressure dressing for 72 hours will prevent enlargment. Application of an ice pack for 30 minutes immediately after insertion also helps. Local irritation, rash, pruritus, and pain occur in 4.7% of users, usually during the first month of use.[29] These problems resolve spontaneously, but itching can be relieved by topical corticoid steroids.

Removal Techniques

Removal of Norplant is a minor surgical procedure accomplished in the office under local anesthesia. As for insertion, the patient should read and sign an informed consent to be filed in her medical record.

Norplant removal times range from 10–60 minutes. Clinicians who are experienced at removing implants require less time and have fewer complications. Practicing removal on a model arm after viewing an instructional video tape makes initial removals faster.

Proper positioning of the implants at the time of insertion is the most important factor influencing ease of removal. If the implants have been inserted with the distal tips (those away from the axilla) far apart or with the implants crossing or touching one another, a larger incision and more instrumental manipulation are required. Removal is easiest when the implants are just under the skin with their distal tips close together in a fan shape.

The fibrous sheaths which form around implants can also make removal more difficult, especially if they happen to be very dense. Pain at the time of removal is slight, and systemic analgesia is not required. The most common cause of discomfort during the procedure is injection of the local anesthetic. Patients may feel pressure or tugging from manipulation of the fibrous sheaths and the implants.

Removal with Instruments. Removal requires 3 small sterile drapes, sterile gloves, antiseptic solution such as povidone-iodine, 18-gauge and 25-gauge 1.5 inch needles with a 5 ml syringe, local anesthetic (1% lidocaine with 1:100,000 epinephrine, buffered with 1 meq sodium bicarbonate per 10 ml lidocaine), one curved and one straight mosquito clamp, 4 x 4 sterile gauze sponges, and a no. 11 blade scalpel.

The patient is placed in a supine position with her arm flexed and externally rotated as for insertion. A thick book positioned under the patient's arm can make her more comfortable and provide a better operating field. A sterile towel is placed under the arm. The implants are exposed by retracting the skin above and below the implants, and the skin is cleansed with the antiseptic solution and draped. The third towel is used to create a sterile field for instruments. A Mayo stand is helpful. Wearing sterile gloves, an incision site is selected by pressing down on the proximal ends of the capsules and palpating their distal tips with a finger. Careful selection of the incision site is critical for easy removal. The best incision site is right at the distal tips, midway between the most medial and lateral implants. This can be the same as the insertion site, but generally the removal incision is made a few millimeters higher up on the arm to ensure placing it as close as possible to the tips of all the implants.

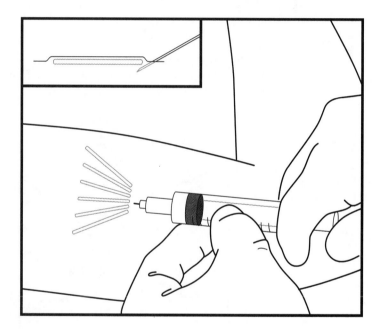

A local anesthetic containing 1:100,000 epinephrine reduces bleeding and allows better visualization of the implants. The 25-gauge needle is used to raise a 1 cm wheal of local anesthetic. Injection of too much anesthetic over the implants can obscure the tips and make removal more difficult. A 3–5 mm incision is made with the no. 11 scalpel. A larger incision is not required and can cause bleeding that can obscure the implants. Sitting on a wheeled stool usually makes the clinician more comfortable.

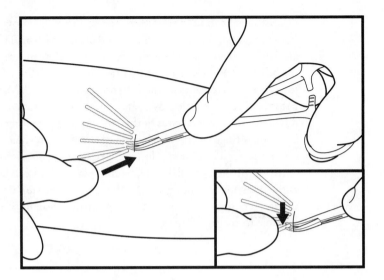

The implant that is most superficial and closest to the incision is removed first. This implant is pushed gently toward the incision with the fingers until the tip is visible and can be grasped with a curved mosquito clamp.

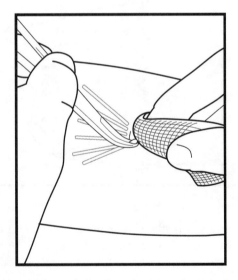

The fibrous sheath is dissected away using a finger covered with an opened gauze sponge. If the sheath is too dense for the sponge, it can be cautiously dissected with the scalpel, taking care not to cut open the implant.

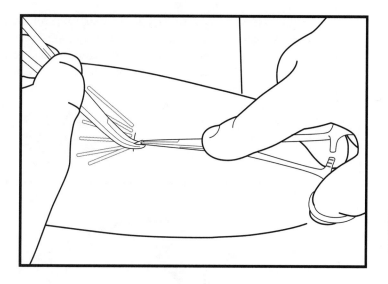

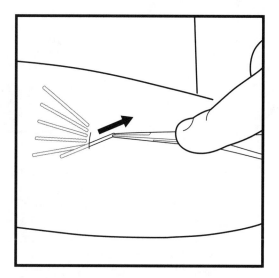

Once the sheath is opened and the tip of the first implant is exposed, it is grasped with the straight clamp. The first clamp is released and the implant is gently pulled out. This procedure is repeated with the remaining implants.

If the implant tips cannot be guided to the incision with digital pressure on the skin above the implants, the jaws of the straight mosquito are inserted into the incision and opened just beneath the skin to separate the tissue layers. The straight clamp is removed, and the curved clamp is inserted with the tips pointing upward toward the skin. The clamp is opened and the implant is guided down between the jaws with a forefinger on the skin above the implant. When the implant is felt between the jaws of the clamp, it is secured at the first or second ratchet. Too much pressure on the implant can fracture the Silastic capsule, making removal more difficult. The implant should not be pulled out with the curved clamp.

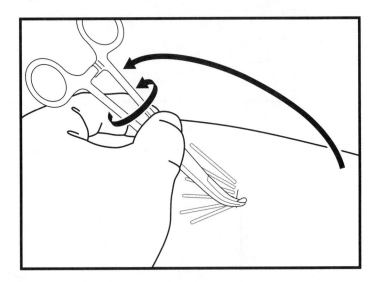

If the implant cannot be seen, after gentle traction, the clamp handle is flipped 180 degrees until it points in the opposite direction, toward the patient's head. The soft tissue surrounding the implant is cleared away with an opened sponge, or if necessary, the scalpel tip. The exposed portion is then grasped with the straight clamp, the curved clamp is released, and the implant is removed with gentle traction. The procedure is repeated until all the implants are removed.

At the completion of the procedure, the implants should be counted to ensure that all have been removed. If any of the implants have been broken, the pieces should be aligned and compared with an intact capsule to determine that all of the implant has been removed. All of the implants should be shown to the patient. An adhesive strip is used to close the incision while pinching the skin edges together. A pressure dressing is then applied as after insertion, and removed the next day.

If removal of some of the implants is difficult, painful, or prolonged, the procedure should be interrupted and the patient should return in a few weeks to complete the removal. The remaining implants will be easier to remove after bleeding and swelling have subsided. A new incision can be made closer to the implants that were difficult to remove the first time. Even if some of the implants remain, the patient should immediately begin to use another method of contraception.

Removal with Fingers Alone. Implants can be removed with less pain and bleeding, and through a smaller incision if the use of instruments is avoided. The amount of trauma and bruising in the surrounding tissues is decreased, the scar is less visible, and the risk of breaking the implants is reduced. The disadvantages of this approach are that it can take longer, and that it may not be sucessful for implants that were poorly aligned or too deep at placement.

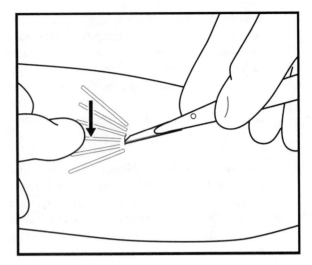

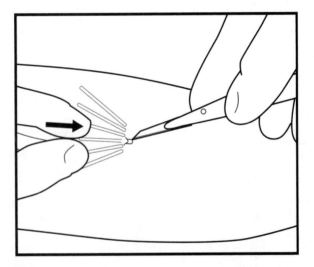

After preparation of the patient, the distal tips of the implants are palpated to identify the implant which is most centrally located and equidistant from the other tips. Pressure is applied with fingers on the proximal end of the selected implant. A 2–3 mm incision is made at its distal tip. Finger pressure is maintained to better position the end of the implant in the incision. The tip of the no. 11 scalpel blade is inserted into the incision until it touches the sliastic plug at the end of the implant. The fibrous sheath surrounding the implant is then incised by nicking it with the tip of the scalpel blade against the implant plug.

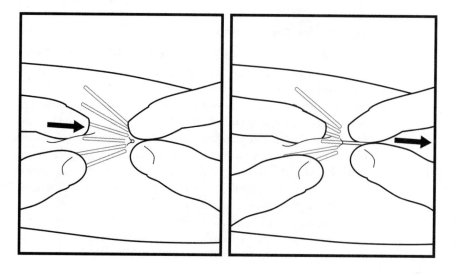

As the sheath is opened, the end of the implant will come into view. With finger pressure on its other end, the implant can be pushed through the incision until it can be grasped and pulled out. The remaining implants can be removed using the same technique if they are not deep or far from the incision. The incision is closed with an adhesive strip and covered with an adhesive dressing. A pressure dressing is not required with this technique because there is little subcutaneous trauma.

Special Attention. Removal is more difficult if the implants are broken during attempts to extract them. Once the capsule is damaged, the implant can fracture repeatedly with further attempts to grasp it with clamps. To decrease this risk, the implants should be grasped by the silastic plugs at their ends and as little traction as possible should be used for exposure and removal. If the scalpel is required to open the fibrous sheath around the implant, care should be taken to avoid slicing the capsule. If it has not been possible to grasp the sliastic plug when opening the fibrous sheath along the length of the implant, cut longitudinally, not across, the implant. Rarely, removal of cut or broken implants will require an additional incision at the proximal end of the implant so that the remaining piece can be removed. Even more rarely, an implant can neither be palpated under the skin nor found through an incision. Such "lost" implants are most easily located with high resolution, short focus ultrasound used during the removal procedure to help place the incision directly over the implant. Radiography will identify implants, but it is not necessary for removal.

Reasons for Termination

Bothersome side effects such as menstrual changes, headache, or weight change are primary reasons for termination of implant use. Desiring pregnancy is the most common personal reason for removal. Menstrual changes are the most common cause for discontinuation of Norplant in the first year of use. The next most common reasons for discontinuing Norplant are headache, weight change, mood change, anxiety or nervousness, depression, ovarian cyst formation, and lower abdominal pain. Headache and weight change are the most frequent, accounting for about 20% of removals for each.[3,12] Presence of ovarian cysts is not usually an indication for removal of Norplant and is almost never a reason for surgery. Most will resolve spontaneously within 4 weeks. Skin conditions, including rashes, dermatitis, and acne, account for about 0.8% of terminations.

User Acceptance of Norplant

Overall, interview surveys throughout the world have indicated that women perceive sustained-release methods, Norplant in particular, as highly acceptable methods of contraception. The most popular feature of Norplant is the ease of use. About 20% of U.S. patients report that friends and relatives notice their implants. This may be a greater problem in warmer climates with less encompassing clothing. Only 25% of the women who report that the implants were noticed were bothered by this attention.[12]

In the U.S., the primary motivations for Norplant use have been problems with previous contraceptive methods and ease of Norplant use. Although fear of pain during Norplant insertion is a prominent source of anxiety for many women, the actual pain experienced does not match the expectations. The level of satisfaction has been high.[12]

Studies of women's attitudes toward sustained-release contraceptives indicate that the great majority of women find them highly acceptable and perceive them as desirable alternatives to conventional contraceptives. Around the world, women who have used Norplant say they have recommended it to friends and would like to use it again.[30-33]

Counseling Women

Because sustained-release contraceptives like Norplant are new in the

U.S., neither the media nor the public have strong opinions about them. Clinicians have an opportunity from the outset to provide sound information and sensitive counseling about these new contraceptives. Frank information about negative factors such as irregular bleeding and possible weight changes will avoid surprise and disappointment, and encourage women to continue use long enough to enjoy the positive attributes such as convenience, safety, and efficacy. Open discussion of side effects will lead to public and media awareness of the disadvantages as well as the advantages of these methods. Helping women decide if they are good candidates for use of Norplant, for example, before they invest too much time and money in this long-acting contraceptive, is a very important objective of good counseling.

Common patient questions regarding Norplant are as follows:

- Is it effective?
- How is it inserted and removed; how long do these procedures take; does it hurt; and will it leave scars?
- Will the implants be visible under the skin?
- Will the implants be uncomfortable or restrict movement of the arm?
- Will the implants move in the body?
- Will the implants be damaged if they are touched or bumped?
- Will this contraceptive change sexual drive and enjoyment?
- What are the short- and long-term side effects?
- Are there any effects on future fertility?
- What do the implants look and feel like?
- What happens if pregnancy occurs during use?
- How long will it take for the method to be effective after insertion?
- Can a partner tell if this method is being used?

General Advantages. One of the major advantages of sustained-release methods is the high degree of efficacy, nearly equivalent to the theoretical effectiveness. In couples for whom elective abortion is unacceptable in the event of an unplanned pregnancy, the high efficacy rate is especially important. There are no forgotten pills, broken condoms, or lost diaphragms. For women who are at high risk of medical complications should they become pregnant, these methods present a significant safety advantage. Users should be reassured that Norplant use has not been associated with changes in carbohydrate or lipid metabolism, coagulation, liver or kidney function, or immunoglobulin levels. Since many women wanting Norplant will have had negative experiences with other contraceptives, it is important that the differences between this method and previous methods be explained.

General Disadvantages. The cost of implants plus fees for insertion total an amount that seems high to many patients unless they compare it to the total cost of using other methods for up to 5 years. Nevertheless, short-term use is expensive compared with the relatively low initial costs of other reversible methods. Sustained-release, progestin-only methods do not increase the risk of developing STDs, but it is not known whether they provide any protection. In women at risk, the additional use of condoms should be recommended. All users must be aware of the possible menstrual changes. It is important to stress that all of the changes are expected, that they do not cause or represent illness, and that most women revert back to a more normal pattern with increasing duration of use.

Cultural factors can influence the acceptability of menstrual changes. Hispanic users of Norplant, for example, are very accepting of irregular or prolonged bleeding.[12] Some religions restrict a woman from participating in religious activity, household activities, or sexual intercourse while menstruating.

Insertion and removal of implants will be a new experience for most women. As with any new experience, women will approach it with varying degrees of apprehension and anxiety. In reality, most patients are able to watch in comfort as implants are inserted or removed. Women should be told that the incisions used for the procedures are very small and heal quickly, leaving small scars which are usually difficult to see because of their location and size.

Prospective users should be allowed to see and touch implants. Women should be reassured that the implants will not be damaged or move if the skin above them is accidentally injured. Normal activity cannot damage or displace the implants. Most women become unaware of their presence.

A few women report sensing the implants if they have been touched or manipulated for a prolonged period of time, or after vigorous exercise. The implants can be visible in slender women with good muscle tone. Darker-skinned users may notice further darkening of the skin directly over the implants; this resolves after removal.

Depo-Provera

The other form of progestin-only, long-acting contraception available in the U.S. is the depot intramuscular administration of medroxyprogesterone acetate (Depo-Provera). It comes as an aqueous suspension in a concentration of 100 mg/ml. The correct dose for contraceptive purposes is 150 mg intramuscularly every 3 months. The effective contraceptive level is maintained for 4 months, providing a safety margin for reliable contraception.

Mechanism of Action. The mechanism of action is the same as with all progestin-only methods, except the circulating level of the progestin is high enough to effectively block the LH surge, and therefore, it is unlikely that any patient will ovulate with this method. Depo-Provera also affects the endometrium and cervical mucus, producing barriers to implantation and sperm penetration, as with Norplant. Suppression of FSH is not as intense as with the combination oral contraceptive, therefore follicular growth is maintained sufficiently to produce estrogen levels comparable to those in the early folllicular phase of a normal menstrual cycle. Symptoms of estrogen deficiency, such as vaginal atrophy or a decrease in breast size, do not occur.

Efficacy. The efficacy of this method is equal to that of sterilization.[34]

Problems. Major problems with Depo-Provera are irregular menstrual bleeding, breast tenderness, weight gain, and depression.[34] The incidence of irregular bleeding is 30% in the first year, and 10% thereafter. After several injections, the majority of women become totally amenorrheic. If necessary, the bleeding can be treated with exogenous estrogen, 1.25 mg conjugated estrogen, or 2 mg estradiol, given daily for 7 days.

Serious weight gain and depression (less than 5% incidence) are not relieved until the drug clears the body 6–8 months after the last injection.

This progestin, in large continuous doses, produced breast tumors in beagle dogs. This is an effect unique to the beagle dog, and has not appeared in other animals or in women after years of use. A very large, hospital-based case-control WHO study conducted over 9 years in 3

149

developing counries has indicated that the risk of breast cancer is very slightly increased in the first 4 years of use, but there was no evidence for an increase in risk with increased duration of use.[35] The results were interpreted to suggest that growth of already existing tumors is enhanced. The number of cases was not large, and the confidence intervals reflected this. For example, the relative risk for ever users (based on a total of 109 cases) was 1.21, but the confidence interval included 1.0, and thus was not statistically significant. Two earlier population-based case-control studies indicated a possible association beween breast cancer and Depo-Provera. One, from Costa Rica, was subject to several biases.[36] The other, from New Zealand, did not find an increased relative risk in ever users, but did find an indication of increased risk shortly after initiating use in early age.[37] These studies have been all limited by very small numbers, and thus have been inconclusive. Certainly the risk, if real, is very slight, and it is equally possible that the suggestions of increased risk have not been free of confounding variables. *It is more appropriate to emphasize that these studies did not find evidence for an increased risk of breast cancer with long durations of use.*

The impact of Depo-Provera on the lipoprotein profile is uncertain. While some fail to detect an adverse impact, and claim that this is due to the avoidance of a first pass through effect in the liver[38,39], others have demonstrated a decrease in HDL-cholesterol and increases in total cholesterol and LDL-cholesterol.[40] The clinical impact of these changes, if any, have yet to be reported.

There are no clinically significant changes in carbohydrate metabolism or in coagulation factors.[40,41]

There is new concern that the blood levels of estrogen with this method of contraception are relatively lower over a period of time compared to a normal menstrual cycle, and therefore, patients can lose bone to some degree.[42] It is unlikely that this bone loss is sufficient to raise the risk of osteoporosis later in life. Furthermore, it is probable that any loss is regained with discontinuation of the method. This concern will require on-going surveillance, especially of past users, but at the present time, this should not be a reason to avoid this method of contraception.

Effect on Future Fertility. The concern that infertility with suppressed menstrual function may be caused by Depo-Provera has not been supported by epidemiologic data. The pregnancy rate in women discontinuing the injections because of a desire to become pregnant is normal.[43] The delay to conception is about 9 months after the last injection, and the delay does not increase with increasing duration of use. Suppressed menstrual function persisting beyond 12 months after the last injection is not due to the drug and deserves evaluation.

Advantages. Like other sustained release forms of contraception, this method is not associated with compliance problems and is not related to the coital event. The freedom from the side effects of estrogen allows Depo-Provera to be considered for patients with congenital heart disease, sickle cell anemia, patients with a previous history of thromboembolism, and women over 30 who smoke or have other risk factors. The absolute safety in regard to thrombosis is mainly theoretical; it has not been proven in a controlled study. However, an increased risk of thrombosis has not been observed in epidemiologic evaluation of Depo-Provera users.

A further advantage in patients with sickle-cell disease is evidence indicating an inhibition of in vivo sickling with hematologic improvement during treatment.[44] Depo-Provera is useful for cases where compliance is a problem, e.g. mentally retarded young women. Another advantage is the finding that Depo-Provera increases the quantity of milk in nursing mothers, a direct contrast to the effect seen with combination oral contraception. The concentration of the drug in the breast milk is very small, and no effects of the drug on infant growth and development have been observed.[45] Depo-Provera should be considered in patients with seizure disorders; an improvement in seizure control can be achieved probably because of the sedative properties of progestins.[46]

Other benefits associated with Depo-Provera use include a decreased risk of endometrial and ovarian cancer[35,47], and probably the same benefits associated with the progestin impact of oral contraceptives: reduced menstrual flow and anemia, less PID, less endometriosis, fewer uterine fibroids, and fewer ectopic pregnancies.

Norethindrone Enanthate

Norethindrone enanthate is given in a dose of 200 mg intramuscularly every 2 months.[47] This progestin acts in the same way as Depo-Provera, and has the same problems.

References

1. Segal SJ, A new delivery system for contraceptive steroids, Am J Obstet Gynecol 157:1090, 1987.

2. Roy S, Mishell DR Jr, Robertson D, Krauss RM, Lacarra M, Duda MJ, Long-term reversible contraception with levonorgestrel-releasing Silastic rods, Am J Obstet Gynecol 148:1006, 1984.

3. Sivin I, International experience with Norplant and Norplant-2 contraceptives, Stud Fam Plann 19:81, 1988.

4. Trussell J, Hatcher RA, Cates W Jr, Stewart FH, Kost K, Contraceptive failure in the United States: An update, Stud Fam Plann 21:51, 1990.

5. Croxatto HB, Diaz S, Pavez M, Clinical chemistry in women treated with progestogen implants, Contraception 18:441, 1978.

6. Brache V, Faundes A, Johansson E, Alvarez F, Anovulation, inadequate luteal phase, and poor sperm penetration in cervical mucus during prolonged use of Norplant implants, Contraception 31:261, 1985.

7. Brache V, Alvarez-Sanchez F, Faundes A, Tejada AS, Cochon L, Ovarian endocrine function through five years of continuous treatment with Norplant subdermal contraceptive implants, Contraception 41:169, 1990.

8. Affandi B, Cekan S, Boonkasemanti R, Samil RS, Dicsfalusy E, The interaction between sex hormone binding globulin and levonorgestrel released from Norplant, an implantable contraceptive, Contraception 35:135, 1987.

9. Alvarez F, Brache V, Tejada AS, Faundes A, Abnormal endocrine profile among women with confirmed or presumed ovulation during long-term Norplant use, Contraception 33:111, 1986.

10. Croxatto HB, Diaz S, Salvatierra AM, Morales P, Ebensperger C, Brandeis A, Treatment with Norplant subdermal implants inhibits sperm penetration through cervical mucus in vitro, Contraception 36:193, 1987.

11. Segal SJ, Alvarez-Sanchez F, Brache V, Faundes A, Vilja P, Tuohimaa P, Norplant implants: The mechanism of contraceptive action, Fertil Steril 56:273, 1991.

12. Darney PD, Atkinson E, Tanner ST, MacPherson S, Hellerstein S, Alvarado AM, Acceptance and perceptions of Norplant among users in San Francisco, USA, Stud Fam Plann 21:152, 1990.

13. Darney PD, Klaisle CM, Tanner ST, Alvarado AM, Sustained release contraceptives, Curr Prob Obstet Gynecol Fertil 13:87, 1990.

14. Centers for Disease Control, Ectopic pregnancy in the United States, 1970–1988, CDC Surveillance Summaries, MMWR 38:1, 1989.

15. Franks AL, Beral V, Cates W Jr, Hogue CJ, Contraception and ectopic pregnancy risk, Am J Obstet Gynecol 163:1120, 1990.

16. Sivin I, Alvarez-Sanchez F, Diaz S, Holma P, Coutinho E, McDonald O, Robertson DN, Stern J, Three-year experience with Norplant subdermal contraception, Fertil Steril 39:799, 1983.

17. Shoupe D, Mishell DR Jr, Bopp B, Fiedling M, The significance of bleeding patterns in Norplant implant users, Obstet Gynecol 77:256, 1991.

18. Nilsson C, Holma P, Menstrual blood loss with contraceptive subdermal levonorgestrel implants, Fertil Steril 35:304, 1981.

19. Fakeye O, Balogh S, Effect of Norplant contraceptive use on hemoglobin, packed cell volume, and menstrual bleeding patterns, Contraception 39:265, 1989.

20. Diaz S, Croxatto HB, Pavez M, Belhadj H, Stern J, Sivin I, Clinical assessment of treatments for prolonged bleeding in users of Norplant implants, Contraception 42:97, 1990.

21. Croxatto HB, Diaz S, Robertson D, Pavez M, Clinical chemistries in women treated with levonorgestrel implant (Norplant) or a TCu 200 IUD, Contraception 27:281, 1983.

22. Konje JC, Otolorin EO, Ladipo OA, Changes in carbohydrate metabolism during 30 months on Norplant, Contraception 44:163, 1991.

23. Shaaban MM, Elwan SI, El-Sharkawy MM, Farghaly AS, Effect of subdermal lenonorgestrel contraceptive implants, Norplant, on liver functions, Contraception 30:407, 1984.

24. Singh K, Viegas OAC, Liew D, Singh P, Ratnam SS, Two-year follow-up of changes in clinical chemistry in Singaporean Norplant acceptors: Metabolic changes, Contraception 39:129, 1989.

25. Shaaban MM, Elwan SI, El-Kabsh MY, Farghaly SA, Thabet N, Effect of levonorgestrel contraceptive implants, Norplant, on bleeding and coagulation, Contraception 30:421, 1984.

26. Abdulla K, Elwan SI, Salem HS, Shaaban MM, Effect of early postpartum use of the contraceptive implants, Norplant, on the serum levels of immunoglobulin of the mothers and their breastfed infants, Contraception 32:261, 1985.

27. Bayad M, Ibrahim I, Fayad M, et al, Serum corisol in women users of subdermal levonorgestrel implants, Contracept Deliv Syst 4:133, 1983.

28. Shaaban MM, Elwan SI, Abdalla SA, Dawish HA, Effect of subdermal levonorgestrel contraceptive implants, Norplant, on serum lipids, Contraception 30:413, 1984.

29. Klavon SL, Grubb G, Insertion site complications during the first year of Norplant use, Contraception 41:27, 1990.

154

30. Zimmerman M, Haffey J, Crane E, Szumowski D, Alvarez F, Bhiromrut P, Brache V, Lubis F, Salah M, Shaaban MM, Shawly B, Sidiip S, Assessing the acceptability of Norplant implants in four countries: Findings from focus group research, Stud Fam Plann 21:92, 1990.

31. Gao J, Wang SL, Wu SC, Sun BL, Allonen H, Luukkainen T, Comparison of the clinical performance, contraceptive efficacy and acceptability of levonorgestrel-releasing IUD and Norplant implants in China, Contraception 41:485, 1990.

32. Bashayake S, Thapa S, Balogh A, Evaluation of safety, efficacy, and acceptability of Norplant implants in Sri Lanka, Stud Fam Plann 19:39, 1988.

33. Salah M, Ahmed A, Abo-Eloyoun M, Shaaban MM, Five-year experience with Norplant implants in Assiut, Egypt, Contraception 35:543, 1987.

34. WHO, A multicentered phase III comparative clinical trial of depot-medroxyprogesterone acetate given three-monthly at doses of 100 mg or 150 mg: I. Contraceptive efficacy and side effects, Contraception 34:223, 1986.

35. WHO Collaborative Study of Neoplasia and Steroid Contraceptives, Breast cancer and depot-medroxyprogesterone acetate: A multinational study, Lancet 338:833, 1991.

36. Lee NC, Rosero-Bixby L, Oberle MW, et al, A case-control study of breast cancer and hormonal contraception in Costa Rica, JNCI 79:1247, 1987.

37. Paul C, Skegg DCG, Spears GFS, Depot medroxyprogesterone (Depo-Provera) and risk of breast cancer, Br Med J 299:759, 1989.

38. Fraser IS, Weisberg EA, A comprehensive review of injectable contraception with special emphasis on depot medroxyprogesterone aceate, Med J Aust 1(Suppl):3, 1981.

39. Garza-Flores J, De la Cruz DL, Valles de Bourges V, Sanchez-Nuncio R, Martinez M, Fuziwara JL, Perez-Palacios G, Long-term effects of depot-medroxyprogesterone acetate on lipoprotein metabolism, Contraception 44:61, 1991.

40. Fahmy K, Khairy M, Allam G, Gobran F, Allush M, Effect of depo-medroxyprogesterone acetate on coagulation factors and serum lipids in Egyptian women, Contraception 44:431, 1991.

41. Fahmy K, Abdel-Razik M, Shaaraway M, Al-Kholy G, Saad S, Wagdi A, Al-Azzony M, Effect of long-acting progestagen-only injectable contraceptives on carbohydrate metabolism and its hormonal profile, Contraception 44:419, 1991.

42. Cundy T, Evans M, Roberts H, Wattie D, Ames R, Reid IR, Bone density in women receiving depot medroxyprogesterone acetate for contraception, Br Med J 303:13, 1991.

43. Pardthaisong T, Return of fertility after use of the injectable contraceptive Depo Provera: Up-dated analysis, J Biosoc Sci 16:23, 1984.

44. DeCeular K, Gruber C, Hayes R, Serjeant GR, Medroxy-progesterone acetate and homozygous sickle-cell disease, Lancet ii:229, 1982.

45. Jimenez J, Ochoa M, Soler MP, Portales P, Long-term follow-up of children breast-fed by mothers receiving depot-medroxyprogesterone acetate, Contraception 30:5232, 1984.

46. Mattson RH, Cramer JA, Caldwell BV, Siconolfi BC, Treatment of seizures with medroxyprogesterone acetate: Preliminary report, Neurology 34:1255, 1984.

47. WHO, Multinational comparative clinical evaluation of two long-acting injectable contraceptive steroids: Norethisterone enanthate and medroxyprogesterone acetate. Final report, Contraception 28:1, 1983.

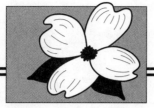

5

The Intrauterine Device (The IUD)

THE GROWING need for reversible contraception in the United States would be well served by increasing utilization of the intrauterine device (the IUD). The efficacy of modern IUDs in actual use is superior to that of oral contraception. Problems with IUD use can be minimized to a very low rate of minor side effects with careful screening and technique. We hope that American clinicians and patients will "rediscover" this excellent method of contraception.

History

A frequently told, but not well-documented story, assigns the first use of IUDs to caravan drivers who allegedly used intrauterine stones to prevent pregnancies in their camels during long journeys.

The forerunners of the modern IUD were small stem pessaries used in the 1800s, small button-like structures which covered the opening of the cervix and which were attached to stems extending into the cervical canal.[1] It is not certain these pessaries were used for contraception, but this seems to have been intended. In 1902, a pessary which extended into the uterus was developed by Hollweg in Germany and used for contraception. This pessary was sold for self-insertion, but the hazard of infection was great, earning the condemnation of the medical community.

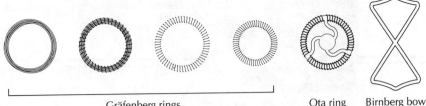

Gräfenberg rings   Ota ring   Birnberg bow

In 1909, Richter in Germany, reported success with a silkworm catgut ring having a nickle and bronze wire protruding through the cervix.[2] Shortly after, Pust combined Richter's ring with the old button-type pessary, and replaced the wire with a catgut thread.[3] This IUD was used during World War I in Germany, although the German literature was quick to report infections with its insertion and use. In the 1920s, Graefenberg removed the tail and pessary because he believed this was the cause of infection. He reported his experience in 1930, using rings made of coiled silver and gold, then steel.[4]

The Graefenberg ring was short-lived, falling victim to Nazi political philosophy which was bitterly opposed to contraception. The non-Aryan Graefenberg was finally sent to jail, but he managed to flee Germany, dying in New York City in 1955. He never received the recognition which was his just due.

The Graefenberg ring was associated with a high rate of expulsion. This was solved by Ota in Japan who added a supportive structure to the center of his gold or silver plated ring in 1934.[5] Ota also fell victim to World War II politics, being sent into exile, but his ring continued to be used.

The Graefenberg and Ota rings were essentially forgotten by the rest of the world throughout the World War II period. An awareness of the explosion in population and its impact began to grow in the first two decades after World War II. In 1959, reports from Japan and Israel by Ishihama and Oppenheimer once again stirred interest in the rings.[6,7] The Oppenheimer report was in the American Journal of Obstetrics and Gynecology, and several American gynecologists were stimulated to use rings of silver or silk, and others to develop their own devices.

In the 1960s and 1970s, the IUD thrived. Techniques were modified and a plethora of types introduced. The various devices developed in the 1960s were made of plastic (polyethylene) impregnated with barium sulfate so that they would be visible on an x-ray. The Margulies Coil, developed by Lazer Margulies in 1960 at Mt. Sinai Hospital in New York City, was the first plastic device with a memory, allowing the use of an inserter and reconfiguration of the shape when it was expelled into the uterus. The Coil was a large device (sure to cause cramping and bleeding) and its hard plastic tail proved risky for the male partner.

In 1962, the Population Council, at the suggestion of Alan Guttmacher who that year became president of the Planned Parenthood Federation of America, organized the first international conference on IUDs in New York City. It was at this conference that Jack Lippes of Buffalo presented experience with his device, which fortunately as we will see, had a single filament thread as a tail. The Margulies Coil was rapidly replaced by the Lippes Loop, which quickly became the most widely prescribed IUD in the United States in the 1970s.

The 1962 conference also led to the organization of a program established by the Population Council, under the direction of Christopher Tietze, to evaluate IUDs, the Cooperative Statistical Program. The Ninth Progress Report in 1970 was a landmark comparison of efficacy and problems with the various IUDs being used.[8]

Many other devices came along, but with the exception of the four sizes of Lippes' Loops and the two Saf-T-Coils, they had limited use. Stainless steel devices incorporating springs were designed to compress for easy insertion, but the movement of these devices allowed them to embed in the uterus, making them too difficult to remove. The Majzlin Spring is a memorable example.

The Dalkon Shield was introduced in 1970. Within 3 years, a high incidence of pelvic infection was recognized. There is no doubt that the problems with the Dalkon Shield were due to defective construction, pointed out as early as 1975 by Tatum.[9] The multifilamented tail (hundreds of fibers enclosed in a sheath) of the Dalkon Shield provided a pathway for bacteria to ascend protected from the barrier of cervical mucus.

Although sales were discontinued in 1975, a call for removal of all Dalkon Shields was not issued until the early 1980s. The large number of women with pelvic infections led to many lawsuits against the pharmaceutical company, ultimately causing its bankruptcy. Unfortunately, the Dalkon Shield problem tainted all IUDs and ever since, media and the public have inappropriately regarded all IUDs in a single, generic fashion.

About the time of the introduction of the Dalkon Shield, the U.S. Senate conducted hearings on the safety of oral contraception. Young women who were discouraged from using oral contraceptives following these hearings turned to IUDs, principally the Dalkon Shield which was promoted as suitable for nulliparous women. Changes in sexual behavior in the 1960s and 1970s, and failure to use protective contraception (condoms and oral contraceptives), led to an epidemic of sexually transmitted diseases (STDs) and pelvic inflammatory disease (PID) for which IUDs were held partially responsible.[10]

The first epidemiologic studies of the relationship between IUDs and PID used as controls women who depended on oral contraception or barrier methods, and who were, therefore, at reduced risk of PID compared to non-contraceptors and IUD users.[11,12] In addition these first studies failed to control for the characteristics of sexual behavior which are now accepted as risk factors for PID (multiple partners, early age at first intercourse, and increased frequency of intercourse).[13] The Dalkon Shield magnified the risk attributed to IUDs because its high failure rate in young women who were already at risk of STDs led to septic spontaneous abortions and, in some cases, death.[14] Reports of these events led the American public to regard all IUDs as dangerous, including those which, unlike the Dalkon Shield, had undergone extensive clinical trials and post-marketing surveillance.

The 1980s saw the decline of IUD use in the United States as manufacturers discontinued marketing in response to the burden of litigation. Despite the fact that most of the lawsuits against the copper devices were won by the manufacturer, the cost of the defense combined with declining use affected the financial return. It should be emphasized that this action was the result of corporate business decisions related to concerns for profit and liability, not for medical or scientific reasons. The number of women using the IUD in the U.S. decreased by two-thirds from 1981 to 1988, from 2.2 million to 0.7 million (7.1% to 2% of married couples).[15]

Use of the IUD in the U.S. and the World in 1988 [15, 16]

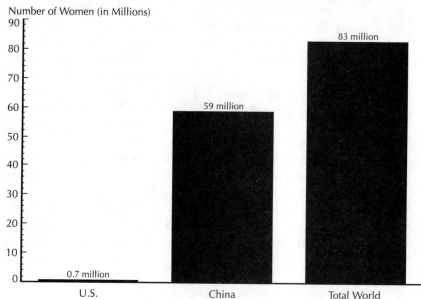

Number of Women (in Millions)

- 0.7 million — U.S.
- 59 million — China
- 83 million — Total World

The reason for the decline in the U.S. is the consumer fear of IUD-related pelvic infection. The final blow to the IUD in the U.S. came in 1985 with the publication of two reports indicating that the use of IUDs was associated with tubal infertility.[17,18] Later, better controlled studies identified the Dalkon Shield as a high risk device, and failed to demonstrate an association between PID and other IUDs, except during the period shortly after insertion. Efforts to point out that the situation was different for the copper IUDs, and that in fact, pelvic inflammatory disease was not increased in women with a single sexual partner[19], failed to prevent the withdrawal of IUDs from the American market and the negative reaction to IUDs by the American public.

Ironically, the IUD declined in the country which developed the modern IUD. It is time for a revival!

The Modern IUD. The addition of copper to the IUD was suggested by Jaime Zipper of Chile, whose experiments with metals indicated that copper acted locally on the endometrium.[20] Howard Tatum combined Zipper's suggestion with the development of the T-shape to diminish the uterine reaction to the structural frame, and produced the copper-T. The first copper IUD had copper wire wound around the straight shaft of the T, the TCu-200 (200 mm² of exposed copper wire), also known as the Tatum-T.[21] Tatum's reasoning was that the T-shape would conform to the shape of the uterus in contrast to the other IUDs which required the uterus to conform to their shape. Furthermore, the copper IUDs could be much smaller than those of simple, inert plastic devices and still provide effective contraception. Recent studies indicate that copper exerts its effect before implantation of a fertilized ovum; it may be spermicidal, or it may diminish sperm motility or fertilizing capacity. The addition of copper to the IUD and reduction in the size and structure of the frame improved tolerance, resulting in fewer removals for pain and bleeding.

The Cu-7 with a copper wound stem, was developed in 1971, and quickly became the most popular device in the U.S. Both the Cu-7 and the Tatum-T were withdrawn from the U.S. market in 1986 by G. D. Searle and Company.

IUD development continued, however. More copper was added by Population Council investigators, leading to the TCu-380A (380 mm² of exposed copper surface area—copper wound around the stem plus a copper sleeve on each horizontal arm).[22] Making the copper solid and tubular increased effectiveness and the lifespan of the IUD. It has been in use in more than 30 countries since 1982, and in 1988, it was marketed in the U.S. by the GynoPharma Corporation as the "ParaGard."

The "Progestasert" was developed by the Alza Corporation at the same time that the copper IUDs were developed. This T-shaped device releases 65 μg of progesterone per day for at least one year. The progesterone diminishes the amount of cramping and the amount of blood loss, thus it is especially useful for women who have heavy periods and cramping. The short lifespan can be and has been solved by using a more potent progestin, such as levonorgestrel.

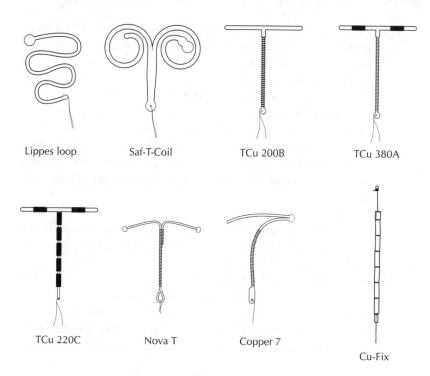

Lippes loop   Saf-T-Coil   TCu 200B   TCu 380A

TCu 220C   Nova T   Copper 7   Cu-Fix

Efforts continue to develop IUDs which address the main problems of bleeding and cramping. The IUDs of the future will probably be medicated with alterations in the frame (size and flexibility).

Types of IUDs

Unmedicated IUDs. The Lippes Loop, made of plastic (polyethylene) impregnated with barium sulfate, is still used throughout the world (except in the U.S.). Flexible stainless steel rings are widely used in China, but not elsewhere.[23]

Copper IUDs. The first copper IUDs were wound with 200 to 250 mm^2 of wire, and two of these are still available (except in the U.S.), the TCu-200 and the Multiload-250. The more modern copper IUDs contain more copper, and part of the copper is in the form of solid tubular sleeves, rather than wire, increasing efficacy and extending lifespan. This group of IUDs is represented in the U.S. by the TCu-380A (the ParaGard), and in the rest of the world, by the TCu-220C, the Nova T, and the Multiload-375. Theoretically, the copper content will provide effective contraception longer than that demonstrated thus far in clinical trials, probably up to 10 years.

The TCu-380A is a T-shaped device with a polyethylene frame holding 380 mm² of exposed surface area of copper. The pure electrolytic copper wire wound around the stem weighs 176 mg, and copper sleeves on the horizontal arms weigh 66.5 mg. A polyethylene monofiliment is tied through the ball on the stem, providing two white threads for detection and removal. The ball at the bottom of the stem helps reduce the risk of cervical perforation. The IUD frame contains barium sulfate, making it radiopaque. The TCu-380Ag is identical to the TCu-380A, but the copper wire on the stem has a silver core (to extend the lifespan of the copper). Its performance is equal to that of the TCu-380A.[24]

Hormone-Releasing IUDs. The only hormone-releasing device marketed in the U.S. (since 1976) is the Progestasert. The Progestasert is a T-shaped IUD made of ethylene/vinyl acetate copolymer containing titanium dioxide. The vertical stem contains a reservoir of 38 mg progesterone together with barium sulfate dispersed in silicone fluid. The horizontal arms are solid and made of the same copolymer. Two blue-black, monofiliment strings are attached at a hole in the base of the stem. Progesterone is released at a rate of 65 μg per day.

The LNG-20, developed by the Population Council, releases 20 μg of levonorgestrel per day. It has been marketed in Europe.[25] This T-shaped device has a polydimethylsiloxane collar attached to the vertical arm, which contains 46 mg levonorgestrel, released at a rate of 20 μg per day. It has been demonstrated to be effective for 7 years.[24]

Future IUDs. Modifications of the copper IUD are being studied throughout the world. The Ombrelle-250 has been marketed in France; it is designed to be more flexible in order to reduce expulsion and side effects. A frameless IUD, the FlexiGard (also known as the Cu-Fix), is undergoing worldwide testing.[26] It consists of 6 copper sleeves (330 mm² of copper) strung on a surgical nylon (polypropylene) thread which is knotted at one end. The knot is pushed into the myometrium during insertion with a notched needle which works like a miniature harpoon. Because it is frameless, it is expected to have low rates of expulsion and removal for bleeding or pain. The TCu-380 Slimline has copper sleeves set at the end of the crossbar that do not rise above the plastic surface of the crossbar, thus facilitating loading of the inserter tube and insertion itself.[27]

Mechanism of Action

The contraceptive action of all IUDs is mainly in the uterine cavity. Ovulation is not affected, nor is the IUD an abortifacient.[28,29] It is currently believed that the major mechanism of action for IUDs is the production of an intrauterine environment that is spermicidal. The protection provided by IUDs against ectopic pregnancy (see below) argues that there exists an extrauterine action as well, perhaps a cytotoxic effect on ova or a disruption of tubal function.

Nonmedicated IUDs depend for contraception upon the general reaction of the uterus to a foreign body. It is believed that this reaction, a sterile inflammatory response, produces tissue injury of a minor degree, but sufficient enough to be spermicidal. Very few, if any, sperm reach the ovum in the fallopian tube. Normally cleaving, fertilized ova cannot be obtained by tubal flushing in women with IUDs in contrast to noncontraceptors, indicating the failure of sperm to reach the ovum, and thus fertilization does not occur.[30] If this action should fail, the inflammatory response would also prevent implantation. In women using copper IUDs, sensitive assays for human chorionic gonadotropin (HCG) find evidence of fertilization in less than 1% of menstrual cycles.[31,32]

The copper IUD releases free copper and copper salts which have both a biochemical and morphological impact on the endometrium. There is no measurable increase in the serum copper level. Copper has many specific actions, including the enhancement of prostaglandin production and the inhibition of various endometrial enzymes. Perhaps the overall inflammatory response is intensified.

The progestin-releasing IUDs add the endometrial action of the progestin to the foreign body reaction. The endometrium becomes decidualized with atrophy of the glands. The progesterone IUD probably has two mechanisms of action: inhibition of implantation and inhibition of sperm capacitation and survival. The levonorgestrel IUD also partially inhibits ovarian follicular development and ovulation. Finally, the progestin IUDs thicken the cervical mucus, creating a barrier to sperm penetration.

With the exception of the progestin-releasing IUDs, no major noncontraceptive benefits are associated with IUD use. The progestin IUDs decrease menstrual blood loss (about 40–50%) and dysmenorrhea. Average hemoglobin and iron levels increase over time compared to preinsertion values.

Following removal of IUDs, the normal intrauterine environment is rapidly restored. In large studies, there is no delay in achieving pregnancy, which belies the assertion that IUD use is associated with infection leading to infertility.[33,34]

Efficacy of IUDs

Intrauterine Pregnancy. The TCu-380A is approved for use in the United States for 8 years, however, it has a theoretical lifespan of 10 years.[35] Pending future studies, leaving the modern copper IUD in for longer than 8 years (up to 10 years) means that clinician and patient would have to accept the possibility of a small loss of contraceptive efficacy, although we hasten to add this has not yet been documented. The TCu-200 is approved for 4 years.

The progesterone-releasing IUD must be replaced every year because the reservoir of progesterone is depleted in 12–18 months. The levonorgestrel IUD can be used for at least 7 years, and probably 10.[24] The progesterone IUD has a slightly higher failure rate, but the levonorgestrel device that releases 20 µg levonorgestrel per day is as effective as the new copper IUDs.[24,36]

First Year Clinical Trial Experience in Parous Women [23, 37]

Device	Pregnancy Rate	Expulsion Rate	Removal Rate
Lippes Loop	3%	12–20%	12–15%
Cu–7	2–3	6	11
TCu–200	3	8	11
TCu–380A	0.5–0.8	5	14
Progesterone IUD	1.3–1.6	2.7	9.3
Levonorgestrel IUD	0.2	6	17

The nonmedicated IUDs never have to be replaced. The deposition of calcium salts on the IUD can produce a structure which is irritating to the endometrium. If bleeding increases after a nonmedicated IUD has been in place for some time, it is worth replacing it.

The actual use failure rate in the first year of use for all IUDs is approximately 3%, with a 10% expulsion rate, and a 15% rate of removal, mainly for bleeding and pain. With increasing duration of use and increasing age, the failure rate decreases, as do removals for pain and bleeding.

In careful studies, with attention to technique and participation by motivated patients, the failure rate with the TCu-380A and the other newer copper IUDs is less than one per 100 women per year.[23,37] The cumulative net pregnancy rate after 7 years of use is 1.5 per 100 woman-years.[38] In developing countries, the failure rate with IUDs is less than that with oral contraception. Failure rates are slightly higher in younger (less than age 25), more fertile women.

Women use IUDs longer than other reversible methods of contraception. The IUD continuation rate is higher than that with oral contraception, condoms, or diaphragms. This may reflect the circumstances surrounding the choice of an IUD (older, parous women).

Ectopic Pregnancy. IUDs do not increase the risk of ectopic pregnancy, and offer some protection.[39-41] The largest study, a WHO multicenter study, concluded that IUD users were 50% less likely to have an ectopic pregnancy when compared to women using no contraception.[42] This protection is not as great as that achieved by inhibition of ovulation with oral contraception. Therefore, when an IUD user becomes pregnant, the pregnancy is more likely to be ectopic. About 3–4% of IUD pregnancies have been ectopic, making the actual occurrence a rare event.

The lowest ectopic pregnancy rates are seen with the most effective IUDs, the newer copper devices (90% less likely compared to noncontraceptors).[43] The rate is about one-tenth the ectopic pregnancy rate associated with the Lippes Loop or TCu-200.[43] The progesterone-releasing IUD has a higher rate which, in fact, is about 50–80% greater than noncontraceptors[43], while very few ectopic pregnancies have been reported with the levonorgestrel IUD, presumably because it is associated with a partial suppression of gonadotropins with subsequent disruption of normal follicular growth and development, and in a significant number of cycles (20–30%), inhibition of ovulation.[24,44,45]

The protection against ectopic pregnancy provided by the TCu-380A and the levonorgestrel IUD makes these IUDs acceptable choices for contraception in women with previous ectopic pregnancies.

Ectopic Pregnancy Rates per 1,000 Woman-Years [43, 46]

All U.S. women	1.50
Non-contraceptive users	3.00
Copper T-380A IUD	0.20
Copper T-200 IUD	0.60
Progesterone IUD	6.80
Levonorgestrel IUD	0.20

Side Effects

With effective patient screening and good insertion technique, the copper and medicated IUDs are not associated with an increase risk of infertility after their removal. Even if IUDs are removed for problems, subsequent fertility rates are normal.[47]

The symptoms most often responsible for IUD discontinuation are increased uterine bleeding and increased menstrual pain. Within one year, 5–15% of women discontinue IUD use because of these problems. Smaller copper and progestin IUDs have reduced the incidence of pain and bleeding considerably, but a careful menstrual history is still important in helping a woman consider an IUD. Women with prolonged, heavy menstrual bleeding or significant dysmenorrhea may not be able to tolerate copper IUDs, but may benefit from a progestin IUD.[48] Because bleeding and cramping are most severe in the first few months after IUD insertion, treatment with a nonsteroidal anti-inflammatory (NSAID) agent (an inhibitor of prostaglandin synthesis) during the first several menstrual periods can reduce bleeding and cramping and help a patient through this difficult time. IUDs rarely cause intermenstrual bleeding, and such bleeding deserves the usual evaluation for cervical or endometrial pathology.

Some women report an increased vaginal discharge while wearing an IUD. This complaint deserves examination for the presence of vaginal or cervical infection. Treatment can be provided with the IUD remaining in place.

Infections

IUD-related infection is now believed to be due to contamination of the endometrial cavity at the time of insertion. Infections that occur 3–4 months after insertion are believed to be due to acquired STDs, not the direct result of the IUD. The early, insertion-related infections, therefore, are polymicrobial, derived from the endogenous cervicovaginal flora, with a predominance of anaerobes.

Compared to oral contraception, barrier methods and hormonal IUDs, there is no reason to think that nonmedicated or copper IUDs can confer protection against STDs.[49] However, the levonorgestrel-releasing IUD has been reported to be associated with a protective effect against pelvic infection.[50] Even though the association between IUD use and pelvic infection (and infertility) is now seriously questioned[10,51], women who use IUDs should be those at low risk for STDs by virtue of a mutually monogamous sexual relationship, or users must be counseled to employ condoms along with the IUD whenever they have intercourse with a partner who could be an STD carrier. Because sexual behavior is the most important modifier of the risk of infection, clinicians should ask prospective IUD users about numbers of partners, their partner's sexual practices, the frequency and age of onset of intercourse, and history of STDs.[52] Women at low risk are unlikely to have pelvic infections while using IUDs.[19]

The IUD is not recommended for women who are at increased risk of bacterial endocarditis (previous endocarditis, rheumatic heart disease, or the presence of prosthetic heart valves). *Women with mitral valve prolapse can use an IUD, but antibiotic prophylaxis (amoxicillin 2 g) should be provided one hour before insertion.*

Asymptomatic IUD users whose cervical cultures show gonorrheal or chlamydial infection should be treated with the recommended drugs without removal of the IUD. If, however, there is evidence that an infection has ascended to the endometrium or fallopian tubes, treatment must be instituted and the IUD removed promptly. Bacterial vaginosis should be treated (metronidazole, 500 mg bid for 7 days), but the IUD need not be removed unless pelvic inflammation is present.

For simple endometritis, in which uterine tenderness is the only physical finding, doxycycline (100 mg bid for 14 days) is adequate. If tubal infection is present, as evidenced by cervical motion tenderness, abdominal rebound tenderness, adnexal tenderness or masses, or elevated white blood count and sedimentation rate, parenteral treatment is indicated with removal of the IUD as soon as antibiotic serum levels are adequate. The previous presence of an IUD does not alter the treatment of PID.

Appropriate outpatient management of less severe infections:

> Cefoxitin (2 g IM) plus probenecid (1 g orally), or
> Ceftriaxone (250 mg IM) plus doxycycline (100 mg bid orally), for 14 days.

Severe infections require hospitalization and treatment with:

> Cefoxitin (2 g IV q 6 h), or
> Cefotetan (2 g IV q 12 h)
> Plus doxycycline (100 mg bid orally or IV)
> Followed by 14 days of an oral regimen of antibiotics.

The following is an alternative regimen:

> Clindamycin (900 mg IV q 8 h), plus
> Gentamicin (2 mg/kg IV or IM followed by 1.5 mg/kg q 8 h).

Actinomyces. The significance of actinomycosis infection in IUD users is unclear. There are several reports of IUD users with unilateral pelvic abscesses containing *actinomyces*.[53,54] However, *actinomyces* are found in Pap smears of up to 30% of plastic IUD wearers when cytologists take special care to look for the organisms. The rate is much lower (less than 1%) with copper devices and varies with duration of use.[53-56] The clinician must decide whether to remove the IUD and treat the patient, treat with the IUD in place, or simply remove the IUD. These patients are almost always asymptomatic and without clinical signs of infection. If uterine tenderness or a pelvic mass is present, the IUD should always be removed after the initiation of treatment with oral penicillin G, 500 mg qid for a month. If *actinomyces* are present on the Pap smear of a well woman, the IUD should be removed and replaced with a copper-containing device when a repeat Pap smear is negative.

Pregnancy with an IUD in Situ

Spontaneous abortion occurs more frequently among women who become pregnant with IUDs in place, a rate of approximately 50%. Because of this high rate of spontaneous abortion and the hazard of septic abortion, IUDs should always be removed if pregnancy is diagnosed and the string is visible. Use of instruments inside the uterus should be avoided if the pregnancy is desired, unless sonographic guidance can help avoid rupture of the membranes.[57] After removal of an IUD with visible strings, the spontaneous abortion rate is approximately 30%. If the IUD cannot be easily removed, the patient should be offered therapeutic abortion because the risk of life-threatening septic, spontaneous abortion in the second trimester is increased 20-fold if the pregnancy continues with the IUD in utero. Even if a patient plans to terminate a pregnancy which has occurred with an IUD in place, the IUD should be removed immediately rather than waiting until the time of the abortion, because septic abortion could ensue in the interval. If there is no evidence of infection, the IUD can safely be removed in a clinic or office.

If an IUD is in an infected, pregnant uterus, removal of the device should be undertaken only after antibiotic therapy has been initiated, and equipment for cardiovascular support and resuscitation is immediately available. These precautions are necessary because removal of an IUD from an infected, pregnant uterus can lead to septic shock.

IUD Insertion

Patient Selection. Patient selection for successful IUD use requires attention to menstrual history and the risk for STDs. Age and parity are not the critical factors in selection; the risk factors for STDs are the most important consideration. In addition, there are other conditions which can compromise success. Women who have abnormalities of uterine anatomy (bicornuate uterus, submucous myoma, cervical stenosis) may not accommodate an IUD. The few individuals who have allergies to copper or have Wilson's disease (a prevalence of about 1 in 200,000) should not use copper IUDs. Immunosuppressed patients and patients at risk for endocarditis should not use IUDs.

Preferably, the absence of cervical infection should be established before insertion. If this is not feasible, insertion should definitely be delayed if a mucopurulent discharge is present.

A careful speculum and bimanual examination is essential prior to IUD insertion. It is important to know the position of the uterus; undetected extreme posterior uterine position is the most common reason for perforation at the time of IUD insertion. A very small or large uterus, determined by examination and sounding, can preclude insertion. For successful IUD use, the uterus should not sound less than 6 cm or more than 10 cm.

Timing. An IUD can be safely inserted at any time after delivery, abortion, or during the menstrual cycle. Expulsion rates were higher when the older, large plastic IUDs were inserted sooner than 8 weeks postpartum, however studies indicate that the copper IUDs can be inserted between 4 and 8 weeks postpartum without an increase in pregnancy rates, expulsion, or removals for bleeding and/or pain.[58] Insertions can be more difficult if the cervix is closed between menses. The advantages of insertion during or shortly after a menstrual period include a more open cervical canal, the masking of insertion-related bleeding, and the knowledge that the patient is not pregnant. These relative advantages may be outweighed by the risk of unintended pregnancy if insertion is delayed to await menstrual bleeding.

Technique. After introducing a vaginal spectrum, the cervix is cleaned with chlorhexadine or povidone-iodine. Place a paracervical block by injecting one ml of local anesthetic (1% chloroprocaine) into the cervical lip (anterior if the uterus is anterior in the pelvis and posterior if it lies posteriorly). Inclusion of atropine, 0.4 mg, in the anesthetic will reduce the incidence of vasovagal reactions. After one minute grasp the cervical lip with the tenaculum ratcheting it only to the first position in a slow, deliberate fashion. Use the tenaculum to move the cervix to the patient's right, revealing the left lateral vaginal fornix. Place the needle tip in the cervical mucosa at 3 o'clock, 1–2 cm lateral to the cervical os, and inject about 4 ml of anesthetic, leaving an additional 1 ml behind under the mucosa as the needle is withdrawn. Now deflect the cervix to the patient's left and inject local anesthetic at 9 o'clock in a similar fashion. Wait a full minute before proceeding.

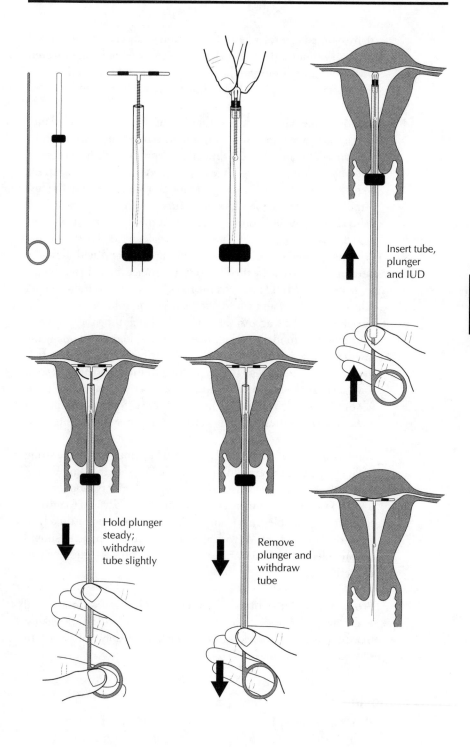

Insert tube, plunger and IUD

Hold plunger steady; withdraw tube slightly

Remove plunger and withdraw tube

Many women can tolerate IUD insertion, especially at the time of menses, without a paracervical block. For some women, however, insertion is less painful with local anesthetic and with administration of a prostaglandin inhibitor one hour prior to the procedure.

Sound and measure the depth of the uterus. The IUD is loaded into its insertion tube immediately prior to insertion. The insertion tube is advanced into the uterus to the correct depth as marked on the tube either by a sliding plastic flange (TCu-380A) or printed gradations (Progestasert). When the insertion tube and IUD reach the fundus, withdraw a few mm. Check to make sure that the transverse arm of the IUD is in the horizontal plane so that the tips of the T will rest in the cornual regions of the endometrial cavity. To release the Progestasert, remove the thread-retaining plug, and withdraw the insertor tube. To release the TCu-380A, advance the solid rod till the resistance of the IUD is felt, fix the rod against the tenaculum which is held in traction, and withdraw the insertion tube while the solid insertion rod is held against the stem of the T, releasing the transverse arms into high fundal position. Remove the solid rod and finally the inserter tube taking care not to pull on the strings. You can ensure that the TCu-380A is in a high fundal position if, after removing the solid rod, you push the insertor tube up against the cross arm of the T prior to withdrawing it completely from the cavity. Trim the strings to about 4 cm from the external os, and record their length in the chart.

Patients with newly inserted IUDs should attempt to feel the string before they leave the examining room. Giving them the cut ends of the string as a sample of what to feel is helpful. Patients should return within 3 months to confirm the presence of the IUD and to provide support, because bleeding changes and expulsion are most likely to occur during this time. As with all office procedures, patients should be provided a 24-hour phone number for urgent questions or concerns.

Prophylactic Antibiotics. Doxycycline (200 mg) administered orally one hour prior to insertion will provide protection against insertion-associated pelvic infection, but it is probably of little benefit to women at low risk for STDs.[59]

IUD Removal

Removal of an IUD can usually be accomplished by grasping the string with a ring forcep or uterine dressing forcep and exerting firm traction. If strings cannot be seen, they can often be extracted from the cervical canal by rotating two cotton-tipped applicators or a Pap smear cytobrush in the endocervical canal. If further maneuvers are required, a paracervical block should be administered. Oral administration of a prostaglandin inhibitor beforehand will reduce uterine cramping.

If IUD strings cannot be identified or extracted from the endocervical canal, a light plastic uterine sound should be passed into the endometrial cavity after administration of a paracervical block. A standard metal sound is too heavy and insensitive for this purpose. The IUD can frequently be felt with the sound and localized against the anterior or posterior wall of the uterus. The device can then be removed using a Facit ureteral stone or alligator type forcep directed to where the device was felt, taking care to open the forcep widely immediately on passing it through the internal cervical os so that the IUD can be caught between the jaws. If removal is not easily accomplished using this forcep, direct visualization of the IUD with sonography or hysteroscopy can facilitate removal. Sonography is less painful and more convenient, and should be tried first.

Fertility returns promptly and pregnancies after removal of an IUD occur sooner than after oral contraception, but later than after using the diaphragm.

If a patient wishes to continue use of an IUD, a new device can be placed immediately after removal of the old one. In this case, antibiotic prophylaxis is advised.

Finding a Displaced IUD

When an IUD cannot be found, besides expulsion, one has to consider perforation of the uterus into the abdominal cavity (a very rare event) or embedment into the myometrium. All IUDs are radiopaque, but localizing them radiographically requires 2–3 views, is time-consuming and expensive, and does not allow intrauterine direction of instruments. A quick, real-time sonographic scan in the office is the best method to locate a lost IUD, whether or not removal is desired.

If the IUD is identified perforating the myometrium or in the abdominal cavity, it should be removed using operative laparoscopy, usually under general anesthesia. If the IUD is in the uterine cavity, but cannot be grasped with a forcep under sonographic guidance, hysteroscopy is the best approach. Both routes may be helpful if an IUD is partially perforated.

Copper in the abdominal cavity can lead to adhesion formation, making laparoscopic removal difficult.[60] Although inert perforated devices without closed loops were previously allowed to remain in the abdominal cavity, current practice is to remove any perforated IUD. Because IUD perforations usually occur at the time of insertion, it is important to check for correct position by identifying the string within a few weeks after insertion. Uterine perforation itself is unlikely to cause more than transient pain and bleeding, and can go undetected at the time of IUD insertion. If you believe perforation has occurred, prompt sonography is indicated so that the device can be removed before adhesion formation can occur.

This problem should be put into perspective. With the new generation of IUDs (copper and medicated), adhesion formation appears to be an immediate reaction which does not progress, and rarely leads to serious complications.[61] In appropriate situations (where the risk of surgery is considerable), clinician and patient may elect not to remove the translocated IUD. However, a case has been reported of sigmoid perforation occuring 5 years after insertion, and the general consensus continues to favor removal of a perforated IUD immediately upon diagnosis.[62]

IUD Myths

We hope the information in this chapter will lay to rest 4 specific myths associated with IUDs. For emphasis, the following sentences provide the correct responses to what we believe are common misconceptions among clinicians:

1. IUDs are *NOT* abortifacients.
2. An increased risk of infection with the modern IUD is related *ONLY* to the insertion.
3. The modern IUD *HAS NOT* exposed clinicians to litigation.
4. IUDs *DO NOT* increase the risk of ectopic pregnancy.

References

1. Huber SC, Piotrow PT, Orlans B, Dommer G, Intrauterine devices, Pop Reports, Series B, No.2, 1975.

2. Richter R, Ein mittel zur verhutung der konzeption, Deutsche Med Wochenschrift 35:1525, 1909.

3. Pust K, Ein brauchbarer frauenschutz, Deutsche Med Wochenschrift 49:952, 1923.

4. Graefenberg E, An intrauterine contraceptive method, in Sanger M, Stone HM, editors, *The Practice of Contraception: Proceedings of the 7th International Birth Control Conference, Zurich, Switzerland,* Williams & Wilkins, Baltimore, Maryland, 1930, pp 33–47.

5. Ota T, A study on birth control with an intra-uterine instrument, Jap J Obstet Gynecol 17:210, 1934.

6. Ishihama A, Clinical studies on intrauterine rings, especially the present state of contraception in Japan and the experiences in the use of intra-uterine rings, Yokohama Med Bull 10:89, 1959.

7. Oppenheimer W, Prevention of pregnancy by the Graefenberg ring method: A re-evaluation after 28 years' experience, Am J Obstet Gynecol 78:446, 1959.

8. Tietze C, Evaluation of intrauterine devices. Ninth progress report of the cooperative statistical program, Stud Fam Plann 1:1, 1970.

9. Tatum HJ, Schmidt FH, Phillips DM, McCarty M, O'Leary WM, The Dalkon shield controversy, structural and bacteriologic studies of IUD tails, JAMA 231:711, 1975.

10. Kessel E, Pelvic inflammatory disease with intrauterine device use: A reassessment, Fertil Steril 51:1, 1989.

11. Eschenbach DA, Harnisch JP, Holmes KK, Pathogenesis of acute pelvic inflammatory disease: Role of contraception and other risk factors, Am J Obstet Gynecol 128:838, 1977.

12. Kaufman DW, Shapiro S, Rosenberg L, Monson RR, Mietinen OS, Stolley PD, Slone D, Intrauterine contraceptive device use and pelvic inflammatory disease, Am J Obstet Gynecol 136:159, 1980.

13. Kaufman DW, Watson J, Rosenberg L, Helmrich SP, et al, The effect of different types of intrauterine devices on the risk of pelvic inflammatory disease, JAMA 250:759, 1983.

14. Lee NC, Rubin GL, Ory HW, Burkman RT, Type of intrauterine device and the risk of pelvic inflammatory disease, Obstet Gynecol 62:1, 1983.

15. Mosher WD, Pratt WF, Contraceptive use in the United States, 1973–1988, Advance data from vital and health statistics; No. 182, National Center for Health Statistics, Hyattsville, Maryland, 1990.

16. Population Crisis Committee, Access to birth control: A world assessment, Population Briefing Paper No. 19, Washington, D.C., 1986.

17. Daling JR, Weiss NS, Metch BJ, Chow WH, Soderstrom RM, Moore DE, Spadoni LR, Stadel BV, Primary tubal infertility in relation to the use of an intrauterine device, New Engl J Med 312:937, 1985.

18. Cramer DW, Schiff I, Schoenbaum SC, Gibson M, Belisle S, Albrecht B, Stillman RJ, Berger MJ, Wilson E, Stadel BV, Seible M, Tubal infertility and the intrauterine device, New Engl J Med 312:941, 1985.

19. Lee NC, Rubin GL, Borucki R, The intrauterine device and pelvic inflammatory disease revisited: New results from the Women' Health Study, Obstet Gynecol 72:1, 1988.

20. Zipper JA, Medel M, Prager R, Suppression of fertility by intrauterine copper and zinc in rabbits: A new approach to intrauterine contraception, Am J Obstet Gynecol 105:529, 1969.

21. Tatum HJ, Milestones in intrauterine device development, Fertil Steril 39:141, 1983.

178

22. Sivin I, Tatum HJ, Four years of experience with the TCu 380A intrauterine contraceptive device, Fertil Steril 36:159, 1981.

23. Treiman K, Liskin L, Intrauterine devices, Pop Reports, Series B, No. 5, Population Information Program, Johns Hopkins University, 1988.

24. Sivin I, Stern J, Coutinho E, Mattos CER, El Mahgoub S, Diaz S, Pavez M, Alvarez F, Brache V, Thevinin F, Diaz J, Faundes A, Diaz MM, McCarthy T, Mishell DR Jr, Shoupe D, Prolonged intrauterine contraception: A seven-year randomized study of the levonorgestrel 20 mcg/day (LNg 20) and the copper T380 Ag IUDs, Contraception 44:473, 1991.

25. Luukkainen T, Allonen H, Haukkamaa M, Lahteenmake P, Nilsson CG, Toivonen J, Five years' experience with levonorgestrel-releasing IUDs, Contraception 33:139, 1986.

26. Wildemeersch D, Van Der Pas H, Thiery M, Van Kets H, Parewijck W, Delbarge W, The copper-fix (Cu-Fix): A new concept in IUD technology, Adv Contracept 4:197, 1988.

27. Sivin I, Diaz S, Pavez M, Alvarez F, Brasche V, Diaz J, Odlind V, Olsson S-E, Stern J, Two-year comparative trial of the gyne T 380 slimline and gyne T 380 intrauterine copper devices, Contraception 44:481, 1991.

28. Sivin I, IUDs are contraceptives, not abortifacients: A comment on research and belief, Stud Fam Plann 20:355, 1989.

29. Ortiz ME, Croxatto HB, The mode of action of IUDs, Contraception 36:37, 1987.

30. Alvarez F, Guiloff E, Brache V, Hess R, Fernandez E, Salvatierra AM, Guerrero B, Zacharias S, New insights on the mode of action of intrauterine contraceptive devices in women, Fertil Steril 49:768, 1988.

31. Segal SJ, Alvarez-Sanchez F, Adejuwon CA, Brache De Mejla V, Leon P, Faundes A, Absence of chorionic gonadotropin in sera of women who use intrauterine devices, Fertil Steril 44:214, 1985.

32. Wilcox AJ, Weinberg CR, Armstrong EG, Canfield RE, Urinary human chorionic gonadotropin among intrauterine device users: Detection with a highly specific and sensitive assay, Fertil Steril 47:265, 1987.

33. Vessey M, Meisler L, Flavel R, Yeates D, Outcome of pregnancy in women using different methods of contraception, Br J Obstet Gynaecol 86:548, 1979.

34. Belhadj H, Sivin I, Diaz S, Pavez M, Tejada A-S, Brache V, alvarez F, Shoupe D, Breaux H, Mishell DR Jr, McCarthy T, Yo V, Recovery of fertility after use of the levonorgestrel 20 mcg/day or copper T 380Ag intrauterine device, Contraception 34:261, 1986.

35. Newton J, Tacchi D, Long-term use of copper intrauterine devices, Lancet 335:1322, 1990.

36. Sivin I, Stern J, Diaz J, Diaz MM, Faundes A, Mahgoub SE, Diaz S, Pavez M, Coutinho E, Mattos CER, McCarthy T, Mishell DR Jr, Shoupe D, Alvarez F, Brache V, Jimenez E, Two years of intrauterine contraception with levonorgestrel and with copper: A randomized comparison of the TCu 380Ag and levonorgestrel 20 mcg/day devices, Contraception 35:245, 1987.

37. Sivin I, Schmidt F, Effectiveness of IUDs: A review, Contraception 36:55, 1987.

38. WHO Special Programme of Research, Development and Research Training in Human Reproduction. Task Force on the Safety and Efficacy of Fertility Regulating Methods, The TCu 380A, TCu 220C, Multiload 250, and Nova T IUDs at 3, 5, and 7 years of use, Contraception 42:141, 1990.

39. Ory HW, Ectopic pregnancy and intrauterine contraceptive devices: New perspectives, Obstet Gynecol 57:2, 1981.

40. Makinen JI, Erkkola RU, Laippala PJ, Causes of the increase in incidence of ectopic pregnancy—a study on 1017 patients from 1966 to 1985 in Turku, Finland, Am J Obstet Gynecol 160:642, 1989.

41. Edelman DA, Porter CW, The intrauterine device and ectopic pregnancy, Contraception 36:85, 1987.

180

42. WHO Special Programme of Research, Development and Research Training in Human Reproduction. Task Force on Intrauterine Devices for Fertility Regulation, A multinational case-control study of ectopic pregnancy, Clin Reprod Fertil 3:131, 1985.

43. Sivin I, Dose- and age-dependent ectopic pregnancy risks with intrauterine contraception, Obstet Gynecol 78:291, 1991.

44. Barbosa I, Bakos O, Olsson S-E, Odlind V, Johansson EDB, Ovarian function during use of a levonorgestrel-releasing IUD, Contraception 42:51, 1990.

45. Bilian X, Liying Z, Xuling Z, Mengchun J, Luukkainen T, Allonen H, Pharmacokinetic and pharmacodynamic studies of levonorgestrel-releasing intrauterine device, Contraception 41:353, 1990.

46. Franks AL, Beral V, Cates W Jr, Hogue CJ, Contraception and ectopic pregnancy risk, Am J Obstet Gynecol 163:1120, 1990.

47. Wilson JC, A prospective New Zealand study of fertility after removal of copper intrauterine devices for conception and because of complications: A four-year study, Am J Obstet Gynecol 160:391, 1989.

48. Andersson J, Rybo G, Levonorgestrel-releasing intrauterine device in the treatment of menorrhagia, Br J Obstet Gynecol 97:697, 1990.

49. Buchan H, Villard-Mackintosh L, Vessey M, Yeates D, McPherson K, Epidemiology of pelvic inflammatory disease in parous women with special reference to intrauterine device use, Br J Obstet Gynecol 97:780, 1990.

50. Toivonen J, Luukkainen T, Alloven H, Protective effect of intrauterine release of levonorgestrel on pelvic infection: Three years' comparative experience of levonorgestrel and copper-releasing intrauterine devices, Obstet Gynecol 77:261, 1991.

51. Kronmal RA, Whitney CW, Mumford SD, The intrauterine device and pelvic inflammatory disease; The Women's Health Study reanalyzed, J Clin Epidemiol 44:109, 1991.

181

52. Lee NC, Rubin GL, Grimes DA, Measures of sexual behavior and the risk of pelvic inflammatory disease, Obstet Gynecol 77:425, 1991.

53. Chapin DS, Sullinger JC, A 43-year old woman with left buttock pain and a presacral mass, New Engl J Med 323:183, 1990.

54. Keebler C, Chatwani A, Schwartz R, Actinomycosis infection associated with intrauterine contraceptive devices, Am J Obstet Gynecol 145:596, 1983.

55. Duguid HLD, Actinomycosis and IUDs, Int Plann Parenthood Fed Med Bull 17:3, 1983.

56. Petitti DB, Yamamoto D, Morgenstern N, Factors associated with actinomyces-like organisms on Papanicolau smear in users of IUDs, Am J Obstet Gynecol 145:338, 1983.

57. Stubblefield P, Fuller A, Foster S, Ultrasound-guided intrauterine removal of intrauterine contraceptive devices in pregnancy, Obstet Gynecol 72:961, 1988.

58. Mishell DR Jr, Roy S, Copper intrauterine contraceptive device event rates following insertion 4 to 8 weeks post partum, Am J Obstet Gynecol 143:29, 1982.

59. Sinei SKA, Schulz KF, Laptey PR, Grimes D, Arnsi J, Rosenthal S, Rosenberg M, Rivon G, Njage P, Bhullar V, Ogendo H, Preventing IUCD-related pelvic infection: The efficacy of prophylactic doxycycline at insertion, Br J Obstet Gynecol 97:412, 1990.

60. Gorsline J, Osborne N, Management of the missing intrauterine contraceptive device: Report of a case, Am J Obstet Gynecol 153:228, 1985.

61. Adoni A, Chetrit AB, The management of intrauterine devices following uterine perforation, Contraception 43:77, 1991.

62. Gronlund B, Blaabjerg J, Serious intestinal complication five years after insertion of a Nova-T, Contraception 44:517, 1991.

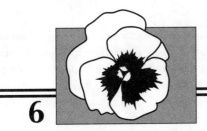

6

Barrier Methods

BARRIER METHODS of contraception have been the most widely used contraceptive technique throughout recorded history. This oldest of methods is now being thrust into the forefront as we respond to the personal and social impact of sexually transmitted diseases (STDs). A new need for sexual safety has brought modern respect to the condom, while the other barrier methods continue to serve well for appropriate couples.

History

The use of vaginal contraceptives is as ancient as homo sapiens. References to sponges and plugs appear in the earliest of writings. Substances with either barrier or spermicidal properties (or both) have included honey, alum, spices, oils, tannic acids, lemon juice, and even crocodile dung. However, the diaphragm and the cervical cap were not invented until the late 1800s, the same time period which saw the beginning of investigations with spermicidal agents.

Intravaginal contraception was widespread in isolated cultures throughout the world. The Japanese used balls of bamboo paper; Islamic women used willow leaves, and the women in the Pacific Islands used seaweed. References can be found throughout ancient writings to sticky plugs, made of gumlike substances, to be placed in the vagina prior to intercourse. In preliterate societies, an effective method had to have been the result of trial and error, with some good luck thrown in.

How was contraceptive knowledge spread? Certainly, until modern times, individuals did not consult physicians for contraception. Contraceptive knowledge was folk knowledge, undoubtedly perpetuated by the oral tradition. The social and technical circumstances of ancient times conspired to make communication of knowledge very difficult. But even when knowledge was lacking, the desire to prevent conception was not. Hence, the widespread use of potions, body movements, and amulets; all of which can be best described as magic.

Egyptian papyri dating from 1850 B.C. refer to plugs of honey, gum, acacia, and crocodile dung. The descriptions of contraceptive techniques by Soranus are viewed as the best in history until modern times.[1] Soranus of Ephesus lived from 98 to 138, and has often been referred to as the greatest gynecologist of antiquity. He studied in Alexandria, and practiced in Rome. His great text was lost for centuries, and was not published until 1838.

Soranus gave explicit directions how to make concoctions which probably combined a barrier with spermicidal action. He favored making pulps from nuts and fruits (probably very acidic and spermicidal) and advocated the use of soft wool placed at the cervical os. He actually described up to 40 different combinations.

The earliest penis protectors were just that, intended to provide prophylaxis against infection. Gabriello Fallopius, one of the early authorities on syphilis, described, in 1564, a linen condom which covered the glans penis. The linen condom of Fallopius was followed by full covering with animal skins and intestines, but use for contraception cannot be dated to earlier than the 1700s.

There are many versions accounting for the origin of the word, condom. Most attribute the word to a Dr. Condom, a physician in England in the 1600s. The most famous story declares that Dr. Condom invented the sheath in response to the annoyance displayed by Charles II at the number of his illegitimate children. All attempts to trace this physician have failed. This origin of the word can neither be proved or disproved.

By 1800, condoms were available at brothels throughout Europe, but nobody wanted to claim responsibility. The French called the condom the English cape; the English called condoms French letters.

Vulcanization of rubber dates to 1844, and by 1850 rubber condoms were available in the U.S. The vulcanization of rubber revolutionized transportation and contraception. The introduction of liquid latex and automatic machinery ultimately made reliable condoms both plentiful and affordable.

Diaphragms first appeared in publication in Germany in the 1880s. A practicing German gynecologist, C. Haase, wrote extensively about his diaphragm, using a pseudonym of Wilhelm P.J. Mensinga. The Mensinga diaphragm retained its original design with little change until modern times.

The cervical cap was available for use before the diaphragm. A New York gynecologist, E.B. Foote, wrote a pamphlet describing its use around 1860. By the 1930s, the cervical cap was the most widely prescribed method of contraception in Europe. Why was the cervical cap not accepted in the U.S.? The answer is not clear. Some blame the more prudish attitude towards sexuality as an explanation for why American women had difficulty learning self-insertion techniques.

Scientific experimentation with chemical inhibitors of sperm began in the 1800s. By the 1950s, more than 90 different spermicidal products were being marketed.[2] With the availability of the IUD and the development of oral contraception, interest in spermicidal agents waned, and the number of products declined.

In the last decades of the 1800s, condoms, diaphragms, pessaries, and douching syringes were widely advertised, however they were not widely utilized. It is only since 1900 that the knowledge and application of barrier methods have been democratized, encouraged, and promoted.

Efficacy of Barrier Methods

Failure Rates During the First Year of Use, United States [3]

Method	Percent of Women with Pregnancy	
	Lowest Expected	Typical
No method	85.0%	85.0%
Diaphragm and spermicides	6.0	18.0
Cervical cap	6.0	18.0
Sponge		
Parous women	9.0	28.0
Nulliparous women	6.0	18.0
Spermicides	3.0	21.0
Condom	2.0	12.0

Risks and Benefits Common to All Barrier Methods

Barrier and spermicide methods provide protection (about a 50% reduction) against STDs and pelvic inflammatory disease (PID).[4,5] This includes chlamydia, gonorrhea, herpes simplex, cytomegalovirus, human papillomavirus, and human immunodeficiency virus (HIV). This protection has a beneficial impact on the risk of tubal infertility and ectopic pregnancy.[5,6] In addition, women who have never used barrier methods of contraception are almost twice as likely to develop cancer of the cervix.[6] The risk of toxic shock syndrome is increased with barrier methods, but the actual incidence is so rare that this is not a significant clinical consideration.[7] Patients who have had toxic shock syndrome, however, should be advised to avoid barrier methods.

Barrier Methods and Preeclampsia. An initial case-control study indicated that methods of contraception that prevented exposure to sperm were associated with an increased risk of preeclampsia.[8] This was not confirmed in a careful analysis of two large cohort prospective pregnancy studies.[9] This latter conclusion was more compelling in that it was derived from a large prospective cohort data base.

The Diaphragm

The first effective contraceptive method under a woman's control was the vaginal diaphragm. Distribution of diaphragms led to Margaret Sanger's arrest in New York City in 1918. This was still a contentious issue in 1965 when the Supreme Court's decision in Griswold v. Connecticut ended the ban on contraception in that state. By 1940, one-third of contracepting American couples were using the diaphragm. This decreased to 10% by 1965 after the introduction of oral contraceptives and intrauterine devices, and fell to about 3% by 1988.

Efficacy

Failure rates for diaphragm users vary from as low as 2% per year of use to a high of 23%. The typical use failure rate after one year of use is 18%.[3] Older, married women with longer use achieve the highest efficacy, but young women can use diaphragms very successfully if they are properly encouraged and counseled. There have been no adequate studies to determine whether efficacy is different with and without spermicides.[10]

Side Effects

The diaphragm is a safe method of contraception that rarely causes even minor side effects. Occasionally women report vaginal irritation due to the latex rubber or the spermicidal jelly or cream used with the diaphragm. Less than 1% discontinue diaphragm use for these reasons. Urinary tract infections are approximately twice as common among diaphragm users as among women using oral contraception.[11] Possibly the rim of the diaphragm presses against the urethra and causes irritation which is perceived as infectious in origin, or true infection may result from touching the perineal area or incomplete emptying of the bladder. Studies also indicate that spermicide use can increase the risk of bacteriuria with E coli, perhaps due to an alteration in the normal vaginal flora.[12] Clinical experience suggests that voiding after sexual intercourse is helpful, and if necessary, a single postcoital dose of a prophylactic antibiotic can be recommended.

Improper fitting or prolonged retention (beyond 24 hours) can cause vaginal irritation or mucosal irritation. There is no link between the normal use of diaphragms and the toxic shock syndrome.[13] It makes

187

sense, however, to minimize the risk of toxic shock by removing the diaphragm after 24 hours and during menses.

Benefits

Diaphragm use reduces the incidence of cervical gonorrhea[14], pelvic inflammatory disease[15], and tubal infertility.[5,6] This protection may be due in part to the simultaneous use of a spermicide.. There are no data, as of yet, regarding the effect of diaphragm use on the transmission of the AIDS virus (HIV). An important advantage of the diaphragm is low cost. Diaphragms are durable, and with proper care, can last for several years.

Choice and Use of the Diaphragm

There are three types of diaphragms, and most manufacturers produce them in sizes ranging from 50 to 105 mm diameter, in increments of 2.5 to 5 mm. Most women use sizes between 65 and 80 mm.

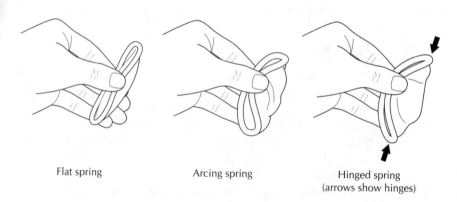

Flat spring   Arcing spring   Hinged spring (arrows show hinges)

The diaphragm made with a *flat metal spring* or a *coil spring* remains in a straight line when pinched at the edges. This type is suitable for women with good vaginal muscle tone and an adequate recess behind the pubic arch. However, many women find it difficult to place the posterior edge of these flat diaphragms into the posterior cul-de-sac, and over the cervix.

Arcing diaphragms are easier to use for most women. They come in two types. The All-Flex type bends into an arc when the edges are pinched together. The hinged type must be pinched between the hinges in order to form a symmetrical arc. The hinged type forms a narrower shape when pinched together. These diaphragms allow the posterior edge of the diaphragm to slip more easily past the cervix and into the posterior cul-de-sac. Arcing diaphragms are used more successfully by women with poor vaginal muscle tone, cystocele, rectocele, a long cervix, or an anterior cervix with a retroverted uterus.

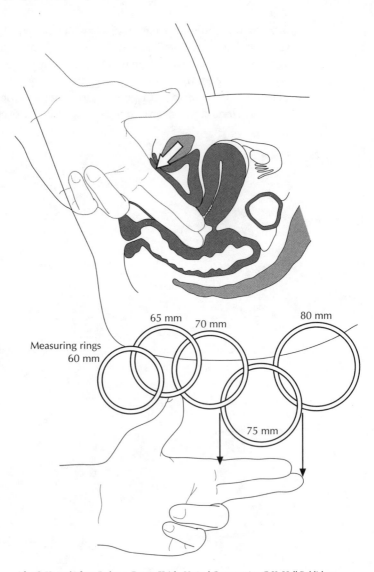

After S. Koperski from **Jackson, Berger, Keith**, *Vaginal Contraception*, G.K. Hall Publishers.

Fitting. Successful use of a diaphragm depends upon proper fitting. The clinician must have available aseptic fitting rings or diaphragms themselves in all diameters. These devices should be scrupulously disinfected. At the time of the pelvic examination, the middle finger is placed against the vaginal wall and the posterior cul-de-sac, while the hand is lifted anteriorly until the pubic symphysis abuts the index finger. This point is marked with the examiner's thumb to approximate the diameter of the diaphragm. The corresponding fitting ring or diaphragm is inserted, the fit to be assessed by both clinician and patient.

If the diaphragm is too tightly pressed against the pubic symphysis, a smaller size is selected. If the diaphragm is too loose (comes out with a cough or bearing down), the next larger size is selected. After a good fit is obtained, the diaphragm is removed by hooking the index finger under the rim and pulling. It is useful to instruct the patient in these procedures as they are experienced. The patient should then insert the diaphragm, practicing checking for proper placement as well as removal.

Timing. Diaphragm users need additional instruction about the timing of diaphragm use in relation to sexual intercourse and the use of spermicide. None of this advice has been rigorously assessed in clinical studies, therefore these recommendations represent the consensus of clinical experience.

The diaphragm should be inserted no longer than 6 hours prior to sexual intercourse. About a teaspoonful of spermicidal cream or jelly, designated for use in conjunction with a diaphragm, should be placed in the dome of the diaphragm prior to insertion. Some of the spermicide should be spread around the rim with a finger. The diaphragm should be left in place for approximately 6 hours (but no more than 24 hours) after coitus. Additional spermicide (an applicatorful) should be placed in the vagina before each additional episode of sexual intercourse while the diaphragm is in place.

Care of the Diaphragm. After removal, the diaphragm should be washed with soap and water, rinsed, and dried. Powders of any sort need not and should not be applied to diaphragm. It is wise to use water to periodically check for leaks. Diaphragms should be stored in a cool and dark location.

Reassessment. Weight loss, weight gain, vaginal delivery, and even sexual intercourse can change vaginal caliber. The fit of a diaphragm should be assessed every year at the time of the regular examination.

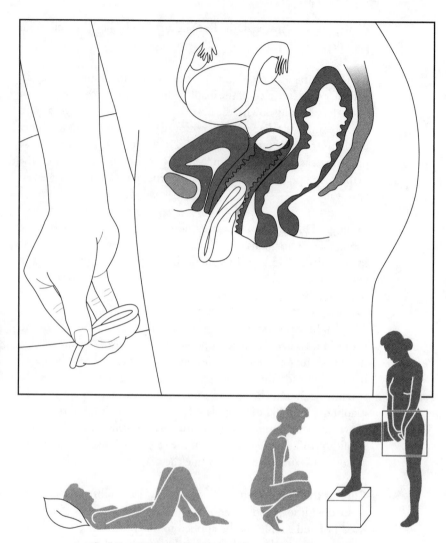

After S. Koperski from **Jackson, Berger, Keith**, *Vaginal Contraception*, G.K. Hall Publishers.

Diaphragm Insertion.

Above: Compression of the diaphragm with the cavity facing upward.

Below: Three commonly used positions for insertion.

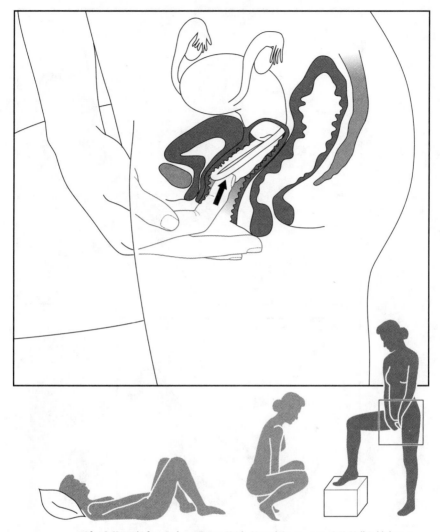

After S. Koperski from **Jackson, Berger, Keith**, *Vaginal Contraception*, G.K. Hall Publishers.

Diaphragm Insertion.

The diaphragm is pushed into the vagina as far as it will go. The leading edge is behind the cervix. The front edge is behind the symphysis pubis.

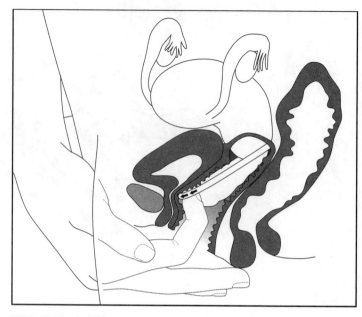

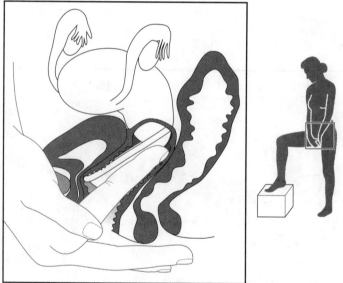

After S. Koperski from **Jackson, Berger, Keith**, *Vaginal Contraception*, G.K. Hall Publishers.

Checking Diaphragm Position.

Above: Checking for forward movement; it should be snug.

Below: Feeling the cervix to make sure it is covered. Move the finger back and forth to feel the rim, then find the bulge in the middle.

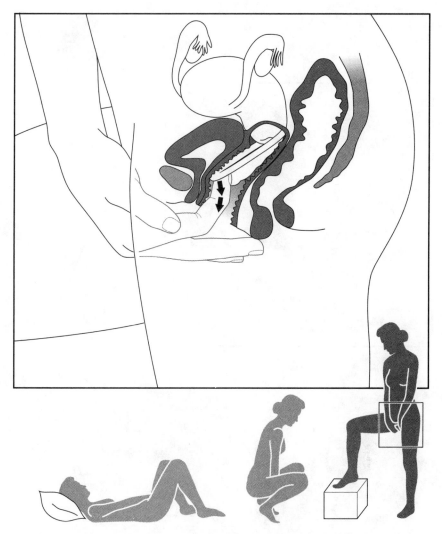

After S. Koperski from **Jackson, Berger, Keith**, *Vaginal Contraception*, G.K. Hall Publishers.

Diaphragm Removal.

Insert the index finger under the front rim and pull downward and outward. An alternative method is to approach the diaphragm with the palm down and insert the finger between the outer edge and the vagina.

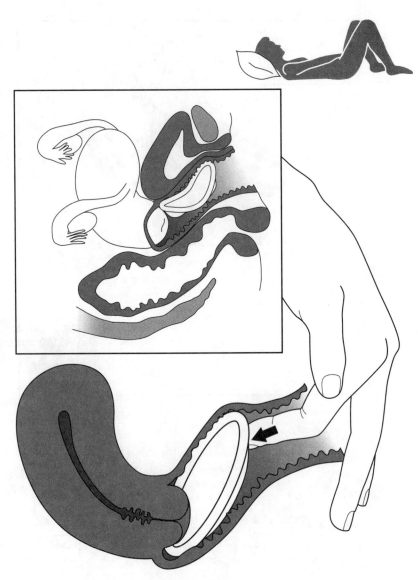

After S. Koperski from **Jackson, Berger, Keith**, *Vaginal Contraception*, G.K. Hall Publishers.

Incorrect Diaphragm Insertion.

Above: The outer rim is correct, but the leading rim is in front of the cervix.

Below: Incorrect placement can be repositioned with a downward push on the outer edge.

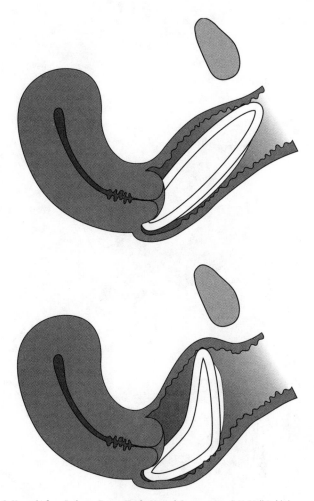

After S. Koperski from **Jackson, Berger, Keith**, *Vaginal Contraception*, G.K. Hall Publishers.

Incorrect Diaphragm Fit (Too Large).

Above: A diaphragm too large cannot fit behind the symphysis pubis.

Below: Forcing a diaphragm which is too large buckles the diaphragm and uncovers the cervix.

198

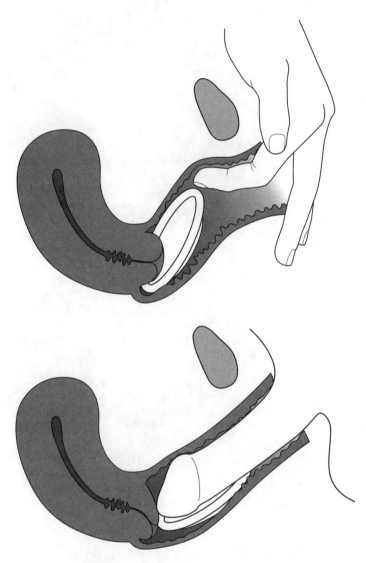

After S. Koperski from **Jackson, Berger, Keith**, *Vaginal Contraception*, G.K. Hall Publishers.

Incorrect Diaphragm Fit (Too Small).

Above: A diaphragm too small does not fit snugly behind the symphysis pubis.

Below: With a diaphragm too small, the penis displaces it and exposes the cervix.

The Cervical Cap

The cervical cap was popular in Europe long before its recent re-introduction into the United States. There are several types of cervical caps, but only the cavity rim (Prentif) cap is approved in the U.S. U.S. trials have demonstrated the cervical cap to be about as effective as the diaphragm, but somewhat harder to fit (it comes in only four sizes) and more difficult to insert (it must be placed precisely over the cervix).[16]

The cervical cap has several advantages over the diaphragm. It can be left in place for a longer time (up to 36 hours), and it need not be used with a spermicide. However, a teaspoonful of spermicide placed in the cap before application is reported to prolong wearing time by decreasing the incidence of foul-smelling discharge (a common complaint after 24 hours).

The size of the cervix varies considerably from woman to woman, and the cervix changes in individual women in response to pregnancy or surgery. Proper fitting, therefore, can be accomplished in only 50% of women. Women with a cervix that is too long or too short, or with a cervix that is far forward in the vagina, may not be suited for cap use. However, women with vaginal wall or pelvic relaxation may be able to use the cap.

Those women who can be fitted with one of the 4 sizes must first learn how to identify the cervix, and then how to slide the cap into the vagina, up the posterior vaginal wall and onto the cervix. After insertion, and after each act of sexual intercourse, the cervix should be checked to make sure it is covered.

To remove the cap (at least 6 hours after coitus), pressure must be exerted with a finger tip to break the seal. The finger is hooked over the cap rim to pull it out of the vagina. Bearing down can help to bring the cervix within reach of the finger.

The cervical cap can be left in place for several days, but most women experience a foul-smelling discharge by 3 days. Like the diaphragm, it must be left in place for at least 6 hours after sexual intercourse in order to ensure that no motile sperm are left in the vagina.

The most common cause of failure is dislodgment of the cap from the cervix during sexual intercourse. There is no evidence that cervical caps cause toxic shock syndrome or dysplastic changes in the cervical mucosa.[17] It seems likely (although not yet documented) that cervical caps would provide the same protection from sexually transmitted diseases as the diaphragm.

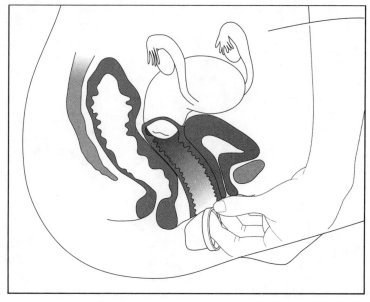

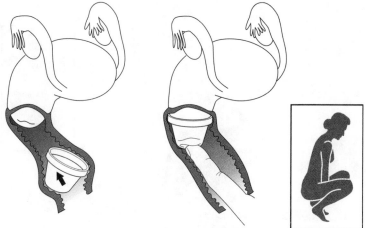

After S. Koperski from **Jackson, Berger, Keith**, *Vaginal Contraception*, G.K. Hall Publishers.

Insertion of the Cervical Cap.

Above: The cap is pushed into the vagina with the index finger.

Below: The cap is pushed onto the cervix, and its position is checked by feeling the cervix through the cap.

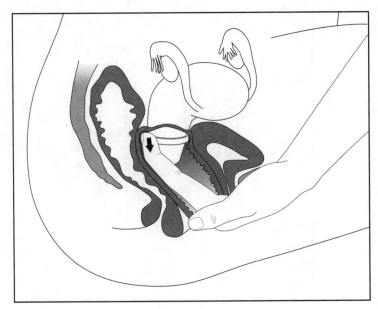

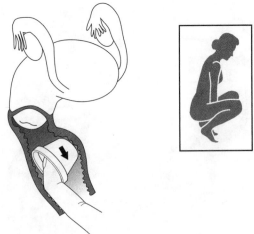

After S. Koperski from **Jackson, Berger, Keith**, *Vaginal Contraception*, G.K. Hall Publishers.

Removal of the Cervical Cap.

Above: The index finger is placed behind the rim, and the cap is dislodged with a downward motion.

Below: The cap is removed by inserting the finger into the cap.

The Contraceptive Sponge

The vaginal contraceptive sponge is a sustained release system for the spermicide, Nonoxynol-9. The sponge also absorbs semen and blocks the entrance to the cervical canal. The "Today" sponge is a dimpled polyurethaned disc impregnated with one gram of Nonoxynol-9. About 20% of the Nonoxynol-9 is released over the 24 hours the sponge is left in the vagina.

The sponge must be thoroughly moistened with water to activate the spermicide. The sponge can be inserted immediately before sexual intercourse or up to 24 hours beforehand. There should always be a lapse of at least 6 hours after sexual intercourse before removal, even if the sponge has been in place for 24 hours before intercourse (maximal wear time, therefore, is 30 hours).

Obviously, the sponge is not a good choice for women with anatomical changes that make proper insertion and placement difficult. In most studies, the effectiveness of the sponge exceeds that of foam, jellies, and tablets, but it is lower than that associated with diaphragm or condom use.[3,18] Some studies indicated higher failure rates (twice as high) in parous women, suggesting that one size may not fit all users.[19]

Discontinuation rates are generally higher among sponge users, compared to diaphragm and spermicide use. For some women, however, the sponge is preferred because it provides continuous protection for 24 hours regardless of the frequency of coitus. In addition, it is easier to use and less messy.

Side effects associated with the sponge include allergic reactions in about 4% of users. Another 8% complain of vaginal dryness, soreness, or itching. There is no risk of toxic shock syndrome, and in fact, the Nonoxynol-9 retards staphylococcal replication and toxin production.

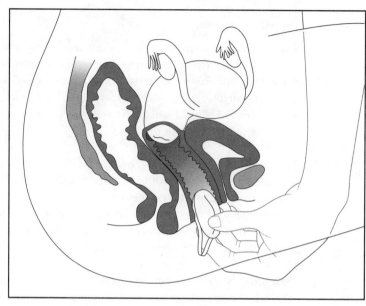

204

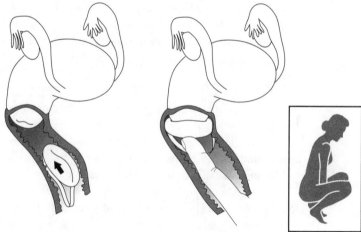

Insertion of the Sponge.

> Above: The sponge is moistened with water (squeezing out the excess), folded upward, and inserted into the vagina.
>
> Below: The sponge is placed firmly against the cervix.

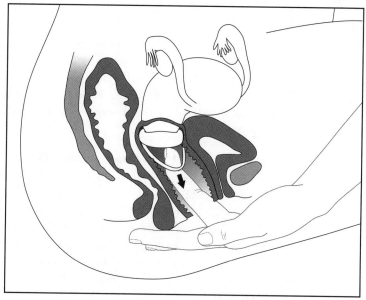

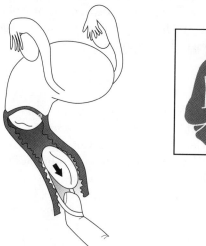

Removal of the Sponge.

The sponge is removed by hooking a finger through the ribbon attached to the back of the sponge.

Spermicides

Jellies, creams, foams, melting suppositories, foaming tablets, foaming suppositories, and soluble films are used as vehicles for chemical agents which inactivate sperm in the vagina before they can move into the upper genital tract. Some are used together with diaphragms, caps, and condoms, but even used alone, they can provide protection against pregnancy.

Various chemicals and a wide array of vehicles have been used vaginally as contraceptives for centuries. The first commercially available spermicidal pessaries were made in England in 1885 of cocoa butter and quinine sulfite. These or similar materials were used until the 1920s when effervescent tablets which released carbon dioxide and phenyl mercuric acetate were marketed. Modern spermicides, introduced in the 1950s, contain surface active agents which damage the sperm cell membranes (this same action occurs with bacteria and viruses, explaining the protection against STDs). The agents currently used are Nonoxynol-9, Octoxynol-9, and Menfegol. Most preparations contain 60–100 mg of these agents in each vaginal application.

Representative Products:

>   Vaginal Contraceptive Film—VCF.
>   Foams—Delfen, Emko, Koromex.
>   Jellies and Creams—Conceptrol, Gynol, Koromex Jel, Ortho Gynol, Ramses, Koromex Cream.
>   Suppositories—Conceptrol Inserts, Encare, Intercept, Prevent, Semicid, Koromex Inserts.

Efficacy

Only periodic abstinence demonstrates as wide a range of efficacy in different studies as do the studies of spermicides. Efficacy seems to depend more on the population studied than the agent used. Efficacy ranges from less than 1% to nearly one-third in the first year of use.[20] Failure rates of approximately 20% during a year's use are most typical.[3] There are no comparative studies to indicate which preparations, if any, are better or worse.

Spermicides require application 10–30 minutes prior to sexual intercourse. Jellies, creams, and foams remain effective for as long as 8 hours, but tablets and suppositories are good for less than one hour. If ejaculation does not occur within the period of effectiveness, the spermicide should be reapplied. Reapplication should definitely take place for each coital episode.

Vaginal douches are ineffective contraceptives even if they contain spermicidal agents. Postcoital douching is too late to prevent the rapid ascent of sperm (within seconds) to the fallopian tubes.

Advantages

Spermicides are relatively inexpensive and widely available in many retail outlets without prescription. This makes spermicides popular among adolescents and others who have infrequent or unpredictable sexual intercourse. In addition, spermicides are simple to use.

Spermicides provide protection against sexually transmitted diseases. In vitro studies have demonstrated that contraceptive spermicides kill or inactivate most STD pathogens, including HIV. However, there is no evidence that spermicides can prevent HIV infection.[21] Clinical studies indicate reductions in the risk of gonorrhea[22,23], pelvic infections[24], and chlamydial infection.[22] There is little difference in the incidence of trichomoniasis, candidiasis, or bacterial vaginosis among spermicide users.[25]

Side Effects

No serious side effects or safety problems have arisen in all the years that spermicides have been used. The only serious question raised is that of a possible association between spermicide use and congenital abnormalities or spontaneous abortions. Epidemiologic analysis, including a meta-analysis, concludes that there is insufficient evidence to support these associations.[26–28] Spermicides are not absorbed through the vaginal mucosa in concentrations high enough to have systemic effects.[29]

The principal minor problem is allergy which occurs in 1–5% of users, related to either the vehicle or the spermicidal agent. Utilizing a different product often solves the problem.

Condoms

Six billion condoms were used world-wide in 1990. However, if condoms had been used in every sex act where they were needed, more than 12 billion would have been used. Although awareness of condoms as an effective contraceptive method as well as protectors against STDs has increased tremendously in recent years, a great deal remains to be accomplished in order to reach the appropriate level of condom use. Contraceptive efficacy and STD prevention must be linked together and publicly promoted.

There are three specific goals: correct use, consistent use, and affordable, easy availability. If these goals are met, the year 2000 will see the annual manufacture of 20 billion condoms.

Two types of condoms are available; most are made of latex. "Natural skin" (lamb's intestine) condoms are still obtainable (about 1% of sales). Latex condoms are 0.3–0.8 mm thick. Sperm which are 0.003 mm in diameter cannot penetrate condoms. The organisms which cause STDs and AIDS also do not penetrate latex condoms, but they can penetrate condoms made from intestine.[30,31] Condom use (latex) also probably prevents transmission of human papillomavirus (HPV), the cause of condylomata acuminata. Because spermicides also provide significant protection against STDs, condoms and spermicides used together offer more protection than either method used alone.

Condoms can be straight or tapered, smooth or ribbed, colored or clear, lubricated or nonlubricated. These are all marketing ventures aimed at attracting individual notions of pleasure and enjoyment. Condoms which incorporate a spermicidal agent coating the inner and outer surfaces logically promise greater efficacy and may reduce STD transmission, but these remain to be determined.

An often repeated concern is the alleged reduction in penile glans sensitivity that accompanies condom use. This has never been objectively studied, and it is likely that this complaint is perception (or excuse) not based on reality. A clinician can overcome this obstruction by advocating the use of thinner (and more esoteric) condoms, knowing that any difference is also more of perception than reality.

As is true for most contraceptive methods, older, married couples experienced in using condoms and strongly motivated to avoid another pregnancy are much more effective users than young, unmarried couples with little contraceptive experience. This does not mean that condoms are not useful contraceptives for adolescents, who are likely to have sex unexpectedly or infrequently.

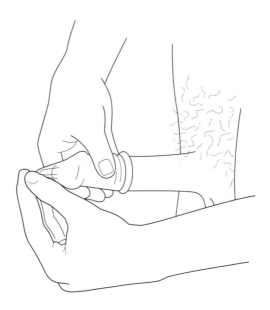

Prospective users need instructions if they are to avoid pregnancy and STDs. A condom must be placed on the penis before it touches a partner. Uncircumcised men must pull the foreskin back. Prior to unrolling the condom to the base of the penis, air should be squeezed out of the reservoir tip with a thumb and forefinger. The tip of the condom should extend beyond the end of the penis to provide a reservoir to collect the ejaculate (a half inch of pinched tip). If lubricants are used, they must be water based. Oil based lubricants (such as Vaseline) will weaken the latex. Couples should understand that any vaginal medication can compromise condom integrity. After intercourse, the condom should be held at the base as the still erect penis is withdrawn. Semen must not be allowed to spill or leak. The condom should be handled gently as finger nails and rings can penetrate the latex and cause leakage. If there is evidence of spill or leakage, a spermicidal agent should be quickly inserted into the vagina.

These instructions should be provided to new users of condoms who are likely to be reluctant to ask questions. Most condoms are acquired without medical supervision, and therefore, clinicians should use every opportunity to inform patients about their proper use.

Inconsistent use explains most condom failures. Incorrect use accounts for additional failures, and also, condoms sometimes break. Breakage rates range from 1–12 per 100 episodes of vaginal intercourse (and somewhat higher for anal intercourse). In a U.S. survey, one pregnancy resulted for every 3 condom breakages. Concomitant use of spermicides lowers failure rates in case of breakage.[32]

Breakage is a greater problem for couples at risk for STDs. An infected man transmits gonorrhea to a susceptible woman about two-thirds of the time.[33] If the woman is infected, transmission to the man occurs one-third of the time.[34] The chances of HIV infection after a single sexual exposure ranges from one in 1000 to one in 10.[35,36]

Condom breakage rates depend upon sexual behavior and practices, experience with condom use, the condition of the condoms, and manufacturing quality. Condoms remain in good condition for up to 5 years unless exposed to ultraviolet light, excessive heat or humidity, ozone, or oils. Condom manufacturers regularly check samples of their products to make sure they meet national standards. These procedures limit the proportion of defects to less than 0.1% of all condoms used.[37] Contraceptive failure is more likely to be due to nonuse or incorrect use.

For the immediate future, prevention of STDs and control of the AIDS epidemic will require a great increase in the use of condoms. We must all be involved in the effort to promote condom use. Condom use must be portrayed in the positive light of STD prevention. An important area of concentration is the teaching of the social skills required to ensure use by a reluctant partner. We believe that bans on condom advertising should be eliminated.

Using scare tactics about STDs in order to encourage condom use is not sufficient. A more positive approach can yield better compliance. It is useful to emphasize that prevention of STDs will preserve future fertility. We would suggest that clinicians consider making free condoms available within their office setting. Manufacturers will sell condoms at a bulk rate, from $50–$100 per 1000, depending upon style and lubrication.

U.S. Condom Manufacturers
Ansell (telephone: 800–327–8659)
Carter Products (telephone: 609–655–6000)
Meyer Laboratories (telephone: 800–426–6366)
Okamoto USA (telephone: 800–283–7546)
Safetex Corp. (telephone: 800–426–2092)
Schmidt Laboratories (telephone: 800–829–0987)

Female Condoms

Female condoms are pouches made of polyurethane or latex which line the vagina.[38] The female condom should be an effective barrier to STD infection, however high cost and acceptability are major problems. Women who have successfully used barrier methods and who are strongly motivated to avoid STDs are more likely to choose the female condom.

References

1. Himes NE, *Medical History of Contraception,* Williams & Wilkins Co., Baltimore, 1936.

2. Gamble CJ, Spermicidal times as aids to the clinician's choice of contraceptive materials, Fertil Steril 8:174, 1957.

3. Trussell J, Hatcher RA, Cates W Jr, Stewart FH, Kost K, Contraceptive failure in the United States: An update, Stud Fam Plann 21:51, 1990.

4. Grimes DA, Cates W Jr, Family planning and sexually transmitted diseases, in Holmes KK, Mardh P-A, Sparling PF, editors, *Sexually Transmitted Diseases,* ed 2, McGraw-Hill, New York, 1990, pp 1087–1094.

5. Cramer DW, Goldman MB, Schiff I, Belisla S, Albrecht B, Stadel B, Gibson M, Wilson E, Stillman R, Thompson I, The relationship of tubal infertility to barrier method and oral contraceptive use, JAMA 257:2446, 1987.

6. Kost K, Forrest JD, Harlap S, Comparing the health risks and benefits of contraceptive choices, Fam Plann Persp 23:54, 1991.

7. Schwartz B, Gaventa S, Broome CV, et al, Nonmenstrual toxic shock syndrome associated with barrier contraceptives: Report of a case-control study, Rev Infect Dis 11(Suppl):S43, 1989.

8. Klonoff-Cohen HS, Savitz DA, Cefalo RC, McCann MF, An epidemiologic study of contraception and preeclampsia, JAMA 62:3143, 1989.

9. Mills JL, Klebanoff MA, Graubard BI, Carey JC, Berendes HW, Barrier contraceptive methods and preeclampsia, JAMA 265:70, 1991.

10. Craig S, Hepburn S, The effectiveness of barrier methods of contraception with and without spermicide, Contraception 26:347, 1982.

11. Fihn SD, Latham RH, Roberts P, Running K, Stamm WE, Association between diaphragm use and urinary tract infection, JAMA 254:240, 1985.

12. Hooton TM, Hillier S, Johnson C, Roberts P, Stamm WE, *Escherichia coli* bacteriuria and contraceptive method, JAMA 265:64, 1991.

13. Centers for Disease Cosntrol, Toxic shock syndrome, United States, 1970-1982, MMWR 31:201, 1982.

14. Keith L, Berger G, Moss W, Prevalence of gonorrhea among women using various methods of contraception, Br J Venereal Dis 51:307, 1975.

15. Kelaghan J, Rubin FL, Ory HW, Layde PM, "Barrier method contraceptves and pelvic inflammatory disease, JAMA 248:184, 1982.

16. Bernstein G, Kilzer LH, Coulson AH, et al, Clinical evaluation of cervical caps, Fertil Steril 38:273, 1982.

17. Gollub EL, Sivin I, The Prentif cervical cap and pap smear results: A critical appraisal, Contraception 40:343, 1989.

18. Edelman DA, McIntyre SL, Harper J, A comparative trial of the Today contraceptive sponge and diaphragm: A preliminary report, Am J Obstet Gynecol 150:869, 1984.

19. McIntyre SL, Higgins JE, Parity and use-effectiveness with the contraceptive sponge, Am J Obstet Gynecol 155:796, 1986.

20. Ryder NB, Contraceptive failure in the United States, Fam Plann Persp 5:133, 1973.

21. Hicks DR, Martin LS, Getchell JP, et al, Inactivation of HTLV-III/LAV-infected cultures of normal human lymponocytes by nonoxynol-9 in vitro, Lancet ii:1422, 1985.

22. Louv WC, Austin H, Alexander WJ, Stagno S, Cheeks J, A clinical trial of nonoxynol-9 as a prophylaxis for cervical Neisseria gonorrhoeae and Chlamydia trachomatis infections, J Infect Dis 158:518, 1988.

23. Austin H, Louv WC, Alexander WJ, A case-control study of spermicides and gonorrhea, JAMA 251:2822, 1984.

24. Kelaghan J, Rubin GL, Ory HW, Layde PM, Barrier-method contraceptives and pelvic inflammatory disease, JAMA 248:184, 1982.

25. Barbone F, Austin H, Louv WC, Alexander WJ, A follow-up study of methods of contraception, sexual activity, and rates of trichomoniasis, candidiasis, and bacterial vaginosis, Am J Obstet Gynecol 163:510, 1990.

26. Louik C, Mitchell AA, Werler MM, Hanson JW, Shapiro S, Maternal exposure to spermicides in relation to certain birth defects, New Engl J Med 317:474, 1987.

27. Bracken MB, Vita K, Frequency of non-hormonal contraception around conception and association with congenital malformations in offspring, Am J Epidemiol 117:281, 1983.

28. Einarson TR, Koren G, Mattice D, Schechter-Tsafriri O, Maternal spermicide use and adverse reproductive outcome: A meta-analysis, Am J Obstet Gynecol 162:655, 1990.

29. Malyk B, Preliminary results: Serum chemistry values before and after the intravaginal administration of 5% nonoxynol-9 creasm Fertil Steril 35:647, 1981.

30. Stone KM, Grimes DA, Magder LS, Primary prevention of sexually transmitted diseases. A primer for clinicians, JAMA 255:1763, 1986.

31. Van de Perre P, Jacobs D, Sprecher-Goldberger S, The latex condom, an efficient barrier against sexual transmission of AIDS-related viruses, AIDS 1:49, 1987.

32. Population Information Program, Condoms, now more than ever, Population Reprots, H-81, The Johns Hopkins University, 1990, p 11.

33. Platt R, Rice PA, McCormack WM, Risk of acquiring gonorrhea and prevalence of abnormal adnexal findings among women recently exposed to gonorrhea, JAMA 250:3205, 1983.

214

34. Hooper RR, Reynolds GM, Jones OG, et al, Cohort study of venereal disease. I. The risk of gonorrhea transmission from infected women to men, Am J Epidemiol 108:136, 1978.

35. Anderson RM, Medley GF, Epidemiology of HIV infection and AIDS: Incubation and infectious periods, survival and vertical transmissions, AIDS 2 (Suppl 1):557, 1988.

36. Cameron DW, Simonsen JN, D'Costa LJ, et al, Female to male transmission of human immunodeficiency virus type 1: Risk factors for seroconversion in men, Lancet ii:403, 1989.

37. Free MJ, Skiens EW, Morrow MM, Relationship between condom strength and failure during use, Contraception 22:31, 1980.

38. Soper DE, Brockwell NJ, Dalton JP, Evaluation of the effects of a female condom on the female lower genital tract, Contraception 44:21, 1991.

215

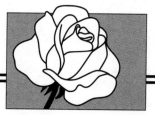

7

Periodic Abstinence

PERIODIC ABSTINENCE as a method of contraception is keyed to the observation of naturally occurring signs and symptoms of the fertile phase of the menstrual cycle. This method must take into account the viability of sperm in the female reproductive tract (2 to 7 days) and the lifespan of the ovum (1–3 days). The variability in the timing of ovulation is the reason why the period of abstinence must be relatively lengthy unless barrier methods are used during the fertile days.

Ovulation occurs at the following median times (note the relatively wide ranges):[1]

- 16 hours after the LH peak (range 8–40 hours).
- 24 hours after the estradiol peak (range 17–32 hours).
- 8 hours after the rise in progesterone (range 12.5 hours before to 16 hours after).

Approximately 1% of reproductive age women utilized some method of fertility timing in 1988.[2] This represented a dramatic decline since the 1960s.[3] This method requires commitment from both partners; it is a way of life. Unsuccessful use can be predicted in couples who are unable to part with sexual spontaneity, women with irregular menses, disorganized people who cannot keep good records, and women with chronic problems of vaginitis or cervicitis.

Methods

Although there are several specific methods, most teachers of periodic abstinence advocate the incorporation of features from more than one method.[4] The sophistication of these methods was made possible by the tremendous increase in the scientific knowledge of the events in the human menstrual cycle. The time of ovulation (the fertile period) was identified in the 1930s, but it wasn't until the 1970s with the advent of the radioimmunoassay, that relatively precise timing of the various events became possible.

The Rhythm or Calendar Method. This method of periodic abstinence was based on the assumption that menstrual cycles were relatively constant, and therefore, the fertile period of the subsequent month could be predicted by the timing of the past cycle.

The general rule is to record the length of 6 cycles, then estimate the beginning of the fertile period by subtracting 18 days from the length of the shortest cycle, and to estimate the end of the fertile period by subtracting 11 days from the length of the longest cycle. Thus a woman with cycles varying from 26–32 days will practice abstinence from the 8th day until the 21st day, a formidable requirement of 14 days of abstinence per cycle. Indeed, because of the normal variation in menstrual cycles, the average couple would practice abstinence 16 days each month.

This method is useful only for women who have relatively regular and consistant menstrual cycles. This method has a pregnancy rate of about 40 per 100 woman-years, and therefore, it is not advocated without combining it with other techniques.

The Cervical Mucus Method. The effectiveness of periodic abstinence has been improved by the development of methods that allow decisions to be made within each cycle. The cervical mucus method is also called the ovulation method, or the Billings method.[5] This method requires sensing or observing the cervical mucus changes over time. A woman successfully practicing this method must become aware of the estrogen-induced changes in cervical mucus which occur at midcyle: an increase in the amount of clear, thin, stringy mucus. Practitioners of this method describe these changes as wet, sticky (but slippery), and moist. This method requires the maintenance of a daily record, at least in the beginning.

The rules for intercourse are as follows:

- Not on consecutive days during the postmenstrual pre-ovulatory period so that seminal fluid will not obscure observation of cervical mucus changes.
- Abstinence when the mucus becomes sticky and moist.
- Intercourse is permitted beginning on the 4th day after the last day of sticky, wet mucus.

The Symptothermal Method. This method utilizes at least two indicators to identify the fertile period, usually combining the cervical mucus method with the basal body temperature (BBT). The BBT is recorded with any thermometer before getting out of bed. Prior to ovulation the temperature is usually below the normal body temperature. It rises about 0.2–0.4° C or 0.4–0.8° F in response to the increasing levels of progesterone after ovulation. The BBT method is so variable that, if practiced alone, it requires abstinence until the night of the 3rd day of a shift in temperature.

Combining the BBT with the mucus method, abstinence begins when the mucus becomes sticky and moist. Intercourse resumes the night of either the 3rd day of a temperature shift or the 4th day after the last day of sticky, wet mucus, whichever is later. Although this method is more complicated, the efficacy is slightly better.

Individual women can be taught to incorporate other signals into their periodic abstinence method. For many women these additional signs and symptoms can add accuracy. These signals include mittleschmerz, breast tenderness, and changes in cervical position and texture.

It is too much to expect the average clinician to provide the necessary instruction and support for these methods. Referral to a local resource is both appropriate and recommended. The local affiliate of the Planned Parenthood Federation of America can direct a clinician to a community program. A directory of all methods and related resources in the U.S., including support groups, is available:

Cooper SA, *Fertility Awareness and Natural Family Planning Resource Directory,* Small World Publications, Corvallis, Oregon, 1988.

219

Most teachers of this method utilize detailed charts for recording changes and signals. The following resources can be contacted for advice, charts, and teaching plans:

Ovulation Method Teachers Association
PO Box 101780
Anchorage, Alaska 99510

Los Angeles Regional Family Planning Council
3600 Wilshire Boulevard
Los Angeles, California 90010

Family of the Americas Foundation
1150 Lovers Lane
PO Box 219
Mandeville, Louisiana 70448

The Couple to Couple League
PO Box 11-1184
Cincinnati, Ohio 45211

Natural Family Planning Program
Center for Life
O'Connor Hospital
2105 Forest Avenue
San Jose, California 95128

Efficacy

The World Health Organization completed a remarkable clinical trial of the periodic abstinence method of contraception in 725 couples in 5 countries: New Zealand, India, Ireland, the Phillipines, and El Salvador.[6-10] The objectives were to determine whether the method could be taught to women of widely different educational and socioeconomical status and to document the effectiveness. 97% of the subjects learned the method well.

The WHO defined failures with periodic abstinence as follows:

- Method-related (pregnancies that occur despite correct application of the rules).
- Inadequate teaching.
- Inaccurate application of instructions.
- Conscious departure from the rules.
- Uncertain.

Among those who learned the method, the pregnancy rate was 22.5 per 100 woman-years, however almost all failures could be attributed to a conscious departure from the rules. Abstinence was necessary for about 17 days in each cycle.

Using the WHO data and a strict application of the definitions for method and use failure, method failure during the first year was associated with only a 3.1% pregnancy rate, but imperfect use with a 86.4% rate.[11] *Thus, if used perfectly, the method is very effective, but all methods of periodic abstinence are extremely unforgiving of imperfect use.*

The probability of pregnancy is greatest when any of the following 3 rules are broken:[11]

- No intercourse during mucus days.
- No intercourse within 3 days after peak fecundity.
- No intercourse during times of stress.

Analysis of the periodic abstinence experience provides these conclusions:[11]

1. Periodic abstinence is associated with good efficacy when used correctly and consistently, but the method is very unforgiving of imperfect use.
2. There is an increased risk of pregnancy during periods of stress.
3. Couples with a poor attitude towards the rules are more likely to take risks.
4. Those couples who get away with taking risks are more likely to take risks again.

A multicenter trial of the cervical mucus method in the U.S. documented over a 2 year period of time a method failure rate of 1.2

221

pregnancies per 100 woman-years, and a user failure rate of 19.3 pregnancies per 100 woman-years.[12]

The cervical mucus method has been compared to the symptothermal method.[13,14] Again, most pregnancies came from conscious departure from the rules. The two methods were comparable, with pregnancy rates of 20–24%.

Couples who do practice periodic abstinence successfully report no significant increase in marital-domestic friction, and some argue that the cooperation and communication required for the use of this method improve a relationship.

Concerns

A lingering concern is that because of periodic abstinence, inadvertent fertilization could occur with aged gametes. Is pregnancy from aged gametes more likely to result in birth defects, spontaneous abortions, and chromosome abnormalities?

No differences have been noted in the frequency of monosomic or trisomic abnormalities in relation to the timing of conception, however conceptions with post-ovulatory aged ova appear to be at increased risk of polyploidy.[15] Furthermore, there is evidence, although not conclusive, to suggest that aged gametes have an increased risk of spontaneous abortions, as well as chromosomal defects.[16] In what is regarded as a well-designed, case-control study, increased relative risks for cleft lip and palate, and congenital hydrocele were associated with periodic abstinence.[17] However, because of small numbers and the very difficult problem of recall bias, it is uncertain if this observation is real or due to chance.

It is worth emphasizing that the well-done and large WHO prospective trial observed no increase in congenital malformations, stillbirths, or spontaneous abortions.[9]

Evidence does support the idea that the further away from the time of highest fertility fertilization occurs, the more likely a male child will be conceived.[18] If this is true, the effect is not great, a ratio of approximately 58 males to 42 females. Here too, the WHO prospective clinical trial failed to detect any difference in the male to female ratio.[9]

Conclusion

In our view, periodic abstinence is best suited for married couples who are united in their motivation to practice this method. With typical practice of the method, the pregnancy rate is about the same as with diaphragm and spermicides. Use of periodic abstinence is possible during lactation, but scrupulous attention is required to detect impending ovulation. It is better to wait until menses resume.

The problem of a long period of abstinence can be overcome by using a barrier method or spermicides during the fertile period. This combination is associated with an efficacy rate that is surpassed only by oral contraception, the IUD, and the sustained release methods.[19]

It remains to be determined whether the various products of advanced technology (self-administered home hormone assays, and electronic instruments with memory to measure temperature or cervical mucus changes) will yield improved pregnancy rates when used in programs of periodic abstinence.

223

References

1. WHO, Temporal relationships between ovulation and defined changes in the concentration of plasma estradiol-17beta, luteinizing hormone, follicle-stimulating hormone and progesterone. I. Probit analysis, Am J Obstet Gynecol 138:383, 1980.

2. Mosher WD, Pratt WF, Contraceptive use in the United States, 1973–88, Advance data from vital and health statistics; No. 182, National Center for Health Statistics, Hyattsville, Maryland, 1990.

3. Forrest J, Fordyce R, U.S. women's contraceptive attitudes and practice: How have they changed in the 80s? Fam Plann Perspect 20:112, 1988.

4. Labbok MH, Queenan JT, The use of periodic abstinence for family planning, Clin Obstet Gynecol 32:387, 1989.

5. Billings EL, Billings JJ, Catarinich M, *Atlas of the Ovulation Method,* 2nd edition, Advocate Press, Melbourne, 1974.

6. WHO, A prospective multicenter trial of the ovulation method of natural family planning. I. The teaching phase, Fertil Steril 36:152, 1981.

7. WHO, A prospective multicenter trial of the ovulation method of natural family planning. II. The effectiveness phase, Fertil Steril 36:591, 1981.

8. WHO, A prospective multicenter trial of the ovulation method of natural family planning. III. Characteristics of the menstrual cycle and of the fertile phase, Fertil Steril 40:773, 1983.

9. WHO, A prospective multicenter trial of the ovulation method of natural family planning. IV. The outcome of pregnancy, Fertil Steril 41:593, 1984.

10. WHO, A prospective multicenter trial of the ovulation method of natural family planning. V. Psychosexual aspects, Fertil Steril 47:765l, 1987.

11. Trussell J, Grummer-Strawn L, Contraceptive failure of the ovulation method of periodic abstinence, Fam Plann Perspect 22:65, 1990.

12. Klaus H. Goebel JM, Muraski B, Egizio MT, Wetzel D, Taylor RS, Fagan MU, Ek K, Hobday K, Use-effectiveness and client satisfaction in six centers teaching the Billings ovulation method, Contraception 19:613, 1979.

13. Medina JE, Cifuentes A, Abernathy JR, Spieler SM, Wade ME, Comparative evaluation of two methods of natural family planning in Columbia, Am J Obstet Gynecol 138:1142, 1980.

14. Wade ME, McCarthy P, Braunstein GD, Abernathy JR, Suchindram CM, Harris GS, Danzer HC, Vricchio WA, A randomized prospective study of the use-effectiveness of two methods of natural family planning, Am J Obstet Gynecol 141:368, 1981.

15. Boue J, Boue A, Lazar P, Retrospective and prospective epidemiological studies of 1500 karyotyped spontaneous abortions, Teratology 12:11, 1975.

16. Gray RH, Kambic RT, Epidemiological studies of natural family planning, Hum Reprod 3:693, 1988.

17. Bracken MB, Vita K, Frequency of nonhormonal contraception around conception and association with congenital malformations in offspring, Am J Epidemiol 117:281, 1983.

18. Kambic R, Gray RH, Simpson JL, Outcome of pregnancy in users of natural family planning, Int J Gynecol Obstet Suppl 1:99, 1989.

19. Rogow D, Rintoul EJ, Greenwood S, A year's experience with a fertility awareness program: A report, Adv Plann Parenthood 15:27, 1980.

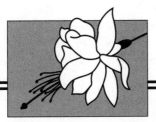

8

The Postpartum Period, Breastfeeding and Contraception

BREASTFEEDING PROTECTS infants against infection, offers an inexpensive supply of nutrition, contributes to maternal-infant bonding, and provides contraception. The relationship between lactation and fertility is an important public health issue. A birth interval of two or more years improves infant survival and reduces maternal morbidity.[1] In developing countries, breastfeeding provides protection from pregnancy and is important for achieving the two-year birth interval.

Giving up breastfeeding was a misguided notion of civilized times. Urbanization, education, and modernization all contributed to a decline in breastfeeding, which, fortunately, has been somewhat reversed. Even in ancient Greek and Roman societies, breastfeeding was disdained by the elite. The tradition of wet nursing (the practice of breastfeeding by someone other than the mother) was popular from the days of the ancient Greeks to the time of medieval Europe.[2] A further decline in breastfeeding came with the introduction of bottle feeding.

The domestication of cattle dates back thousands of years, but the use of animal milk for infant feeding is recent. In the U.S., modification of cow's milk for infant feeding was not established until 1900. In the early 1900s, milk banks were popular, using freezing techniques to keep the milk sterile. But it wasn't until the 1930s that the preparation of infant "formulas" moved from the home kitchen to commercial production and promotion. Breast milk substitutes were initially developed to meet specific needs (allergies and intolerance with cow's milk), but eventually came to be viewed as a means to free women from the responsibility of breastfeeding.

A decline in breastfeeding began in the 1930s (in 1922, about 90% of infants were still being breastfed at one year of age). By the 1950s, the prevalence of breastfeeding on discharge from the hospital fell to 30%, and the downward trend reached its nadir (22%) in 1972.[3] This trend was followed in Europe a decade or two later.

A higher mortality rate in artifically fed infants was observed in the 1900s. By the 1940s, the mortality difference between early and late weaned infants was recognized to be due to conditions of hygiene and general care. In the developed parts of the world, where infants receive good health supervision, the mortality difference is no longer a significant problem. However, in the developing world, excess mortality due to early weaning continues to be high.

The revival of breastfeeding can be attributed to the growth of knowledge regarding the health of infants. The following reasons emerged as motivations to encourage breastfeeding:

1. Breastfeeding has a child-spacing effect, which is very important in the developing world as a means of limiting family size.
2. Human milk prevents infections in infants, both by the transmission of immunoglobulins and by modifying the bacterial flora of the infant's gastrointestinal tract.
3. Breastfeeding enhances the bonding process between mother and child.
4. Breastfeeding protects against breast cancer, especially against premenopausal breast cancer.

Breastfeeding is a personal choice, but one influenced by custom and social and economic circumstances. An increase in breastfeeding has been documented over the last two decades in the U.S., Sweden, Canada, and the U.K.[3,4] Even in the developing world there was evidence of increased breastfeeding. In general, the knowledge that breastfeeding is superior was being spread. But this upward trend in the U.S. peaked in 1982 (at 61% for initiation and 40% for 3 or more months).[3]

Unfortunately, and somewhat perplexing (does it represent more women in the workforce?), is the fact that during the 1980s, there was a steady decline in breastfeeding, reaching 52% for initiation by 1989.[3] By age 6 months, only 19.6% of infants were still breastfeeding. The average duration remains short, usually under 6 months, and most often only 2–3 months. This still provides a significant benefit for the infant, but as we shall see, it is not so good from a contraceptive point of view.

Breast Physiology

The basic component of the breast is the hollow alveolus or milk gland lined by a single layer of milk-secreting epithelial cells. Each alveolus is encased in a crisscrossing mantle of contractile myoepithelial strands. Also surrounding the milk gland is a rich capillary network. Growth of this milk-producing system is dependent on numerous hormonal factors which occur first at puberty and then in pregnancy.

The major influence on breast growth at puberty is estrogen. In most girls, the first response to the increasing levels of estrogen is an increase in size and pigmentation of the areola and the formation of a mass of breast tissue just underneath the areola. Breast tissue binds estrogen in a manner similar to the uterus and vagina, however, the development of estrogen receptors in the breast does not occur in the absence of prolactin. The primary effect of estrogen according to animal studies is to stimulate growth of the ductal portion of the gland system. Progesterone in these animals influences growth of the alveolar components of the lobule. However, neither hormone alone, or in combination, is capable of yielding optimal breast growth and development.

Final differentiation of the alveolar epithelial cell into a mature milk cell during pregnancy is accomplished in the presence of prolactin, but only after prior exposure to cortisol and insulin. The complete reaction depends on the availability of minimal quantities of thyroid hormone. Thus, the endocrinologically intact individual in whom estrogen, progesterone, thyroxine, cortisol, insulin, prolactin, and growth hormone are available can have appropriate breast growth and function.[5]

229

Lactation

During pregnancy, prolactin levels rise from the normal level of 10–25 ng/ml to high concentrations, beginning about 8 weeks and reaching a peak of 200–400 ng/ml at term.[6] Made by the placenta and actively secreted into the maternal circulation from the 6th week of pregnancy, human placental lactogen (HPL) rises progressively reaching a level of approximately 6000 ng/ml at term. HPL, though displaying less activity than prolactin, is produced in such large amounts that it may exert a lactogenic effect.

Although prolactin stimulates significant breast growth, and is available for lactation, only colostrum (composed of desquamated epithelial cells and transudate) is produced during gestation. Full lactation is inhibited by estrogen and progesterone which interfere with prolactin action at the alveolar cell prolactin receptor level. Both estrogen and progesterone are necessary for the expression of the lactogenic receptor, but the sex steroid hormones block the prolactin receptor response.[7,8]

The principal hormone involved in milk biosynthesis is prolactin. Without prolactin, synthesis of the primary protein, casein, and the major carbohydrate, lactose, will not occur, and true milk secretion will be impossible. The hormonal trigger for initiation of milk production within the alveolar cell and its secretion into the lumen of the gland is the rapid disappearance of estrogen and progesterone from the circulation after delivery. The clearance of prolactin is much slower, requiring 7 days to reach nonpregnant levels in a nonbreastfeeding woman. Breast engorgement and milk secretion begin 3–4 days postpartum when steroids have been sufficiently cleared. Maintenance of steroidal inhibition or rapid reduction of prolactin secretion (e. g. with the administration of bromocriptine) is effective in preventing postpartum milk synthesis and secretion.

In the first postpartum week, prolactin levels in breastfeeding women decline approximately 50% (to about 100 ng/ml). Suckling elicits increases in prolactin, which are important in initiating milk production. Until 2–3 months postpartum, basal levels are approximately 40–50 ng/ml, and there are large (about 10–20-fold) increases after suckling. Subsequently, throughout breastfeeding, baseline prolactin levels remain elevated, and suckling produces a twofold increase that is essential for continuing milk production.[9]

Maintenance of milk production at high levels is dependent on the joint action of anterior and posterior pituitary factors. Suckling causes the release of both prolactin and oxytocin.[10] Prolactin sustains the secretion of casein, fatty acids, lactose and the volume of secretion, while oxytocin contracts myoepithelial cells and empties the alveolar lumen, thus enhancing further milk secretion and alveolar refilling. Frequent emptying of the lumen is important for maintaining an adequate level of secretion. Indeed, after the 4th postpartum month, suckling appears to be the only stimulant required; however environmental and emotional states also are important for continued alveolar activity.

The ejection of milk from the breast does not occur as the result of a mechanically induced negative pressure produced by suckling. Tactile sensors concentrated in the areola activate, via thoracic sensory nerve roots, an afferent sensory neural arc which stimulates the paraventricular and supraoptic nuclei of the hypothalamus to synthesize and transport oxytocin to the posterior pituitary. The efferent arc (oxytocin) is blood-borne to the breast alveolus-ductal systems to contract myoepithelial cells and empty the alveolar lumen. Milk contained in major ductal repositories is ejected from openings in the nipple. This rapid release of milk is called "letdown". In many instances, the activation of oxytocin release leading to letdown does not require initiation by tactile stimuli. The central nervous system can be conditioned to respond to the presence of the infant, or to the sound of the infant's cry, by inducing activation of the efferent arc.

The oxytocin effect is a release phenomenon acting on secreted and stored milk. Prolactin must be available in sufficient quantities for continued secretory replacement of ejected milk. This requires the transient increase in prolactin associated with suckling. The amount of milk produced correlates with the amount removed by suckling. The breast can store milk for a maximum of 48 hours before production diminishes.

Suckling suppresses the formation of a hypothalamic substance, prolactin inhibiting factor (PIF). This intrahypothalamic effect is either mediated by dopamine, or, in contrast to the peptide nature of other hypothalamic hormones, PIF is dopamine itself.[11] Dopamine is secreted by the basal hypothalamus into the portal system and conducted to the anterior pituitary. Dopamine binds specifically to lactotroph cells and suppresses the secretion of prolactin into the general circulation; in its absence, prolactin is secreted. Suckling, therefore, acts to refill the breast by activating both portions of the pituitary (anterior and posterior) causing the breast to produce new milk and to eject milk.

Lactation can be terminated by discontinuing suckling. The primary effect of this cessation is loss of milk letdown via the neural evocation of oxytocin. With passage of a few days, the swollen alveoli depress milk formation probably via a local pressure effect. With resorption of fluid and solute, the swollen engorged breast diminishes in size in a few days. In addition to the loss of milk letdown the absence of suckling reactivates dopamine (PIF) production so that there is less prolactin stimulation of milk secretion.

The Contraceptive Efficacy of Lactation

In primitive human societies, the duration of the birth interval has been very important for the survival of the young. Lactation amenorrhea, lasting up to 2 years, has been nature's most effective form of contraception.[12]

Mechanism of Action

Prolactin concentrations are increased in response to the repeated suckling stimulus of breastfeeding. Given sufficient intensity and frequency, prolactin levels will remain elevated. Under these conditions, follicle-stimulating hormone (FSH) concentrations are in the normal range (having risen from extremely low concentrations at delivery to follicular range in the 3 weeks postpartum) and luteinizing hormone (LH) values are in the low normal range. Despite the presence of gonadotropins, the ovary during lactational hyperprolactinemia does not display follicular development and does not secrete estrogen. Therefore, vaginal dryness and dyspareunia are commonly reported by breastfeeding women. *The use of vaginal estrogen preparations is discouraged because absorption of the estrogen can lead to inhibition of milk production. Vaginal lubricants should be used until ovarian function and estrogen production return.*

Earlier experimental evidence suggested that the ovaries might be refractory to gonadotropin stimulation during lactation, and in addition, the anterior pituitary might be less responsive to GnRH stimulation. Other studies, done later in the course of lactation, indicated, however, that the ovaries as well as the pituitary were responsive to adequate tropic hormone stimulation.[13]

These observations suggest that high concentrations of prolactin work at both central and ovarian sites to produce lactational amenorrhea and anovulation. Prolactin appears to affect granulosa cell function in vitro by inhibiting synthesis of progesterone. It also may change the testosterone:dihydrotestosterone ratio, thereby reducing aromatizable substrate and increasing local antiestrogen concentrations. Nevertheless, a direct effect of prolactin on ovarian follicular development does not appear to be a major factor. The central action predominates.

Elevated levels of prolactin inhibit the pulsatile secretion of GnRH.[14] Prolactin excess has stimulatory feedback effects on dopamine. Increased dopamine reduces GnRH by suppressing arcuate nucleus function, apparently in a mechanism mediated by endogenous opioid activity.[15]

At weaning, as prolactin concentrations fall to normal, gonadotropin concentrations increase and estradiol secretion rises. This prompt resumption of ovarian function is also indicated by the occurrence of ovulation within 14–30 days of weaning.

Resumption of Ovulation

The resumption of ovulation in the postpartum period has been well studied in recent times.

Nonbreastfeeding Women. In nonbreastfeeding women, gonadotropin levels remain low during the early puerperium and return to normal concentrations during the 3rd to 5th week when prolactin levels have returned to baseline. In an assessment of this important physiologic event (in terms of the need for contraception), the mean delay before first ovulation was found to be approximately 45 days, while no woman ovulated before 25 days after delivery.[16] Of the 22 women, 11 ovulated before the 6th postpartum week, underscoring the need to move the traditional postpartum medical visit to the 3rd week after delivery.

Breastfeeding Women. In Scotland, no ovulation could be detected in women during exclusive breast-feeding.[17] However, in Chile, 14% of women ovulated during full breast feeding, although full nursing provided effective contraception up to 3 months postpartum.[18,19] It has been argued that the threshold for suppression of ovulation is at least 5 feedings for a total of at least 65 minutes per day

233

suckling duration.[20] However in the studies from Chile, the frequency of nursing was the same in breastfeeders who ovulated and those who did not.

In Mexico, a study of 29 breastfeeding mothers and 10 nonbreastfeeders observed that in the absence of bleeding and supplementary feedings, 100% of the breastfeeders remained anovulatory for 3 months postpartum, and 96% up to 6 months.[21] The median time from delivery to first ovulation was 259 days for breastfeeders compared to 119 days for nonbreastfeeders. However, by the third postpartum month, 18% of the breastfeeders had ovulated.

In a well-nourished population in Australia, less than 20% of breastfeeding women ovulated by the 6th postpartum month, and less than 25% menstruated.[22] Neither time of first supplement nor the amount of supplement predicted the return of ovulation or menstruation. In other words, even in women giving their infants supplemental feedings, there is effective inhibition of ovulation during the first 6 months of breastfeeding.

Risk of Pregnancy

Over the years, Roger Short has done as much as anyone, if not more, to increase our appreciation for the importance of breastfeeding. Now he has documented from Australia that among women who have unprotected intercourse during lactation amenorrhea and use contraception when menses resume, 1.7% become pregnant in the first 6 months of breastfeeding, 7% after 12 months, and 13% after 24 months.[23]

In Santiago, Chile, the probability of pregnancy in breastfeeding women was as follows:[24]

> Amenorrheic women: 0.9% at 6 months; 17% at 12 months.
> Menstruating women: 36% at 6 months; 55% at 12 months.

It is apparent that while lactation provides a contraceptive effect, it is variable and not reliable for every woman, especially in view of the variablity in intensity of breastfeeding and the use of supplemental feeding.

An international group of researchers in the area of lactational infertility reached the following consensus in 1989, called the Bellagio Consensus (after the site of the conference at Bellagio, Italy):[25]

> "The maximum birth spacing effect of breastfeeding is achieved when a mother 'fully' or nearly fully breastfeeds and remains amenorrheic. When these two conditions are fulfilled, breastfeeding provides more than 98% protection from pregnancy in the first six months."

Full breastfeeding means that the infant's total suckling stimulus is directed to the mother. There is no diminution of suckling by supplementation or the use of a pacifier.

Only amenorrheic women who exclusively breastfeed at regular intervals, including nighttime, during the first 6 months have the contraceptive protection equivalent to that provided by oral contraception; with menstruation or after 6 months, the risk of ovulation increases.[26] Supplemental feeding increases the risk of ovulation (and pregnancy) even in amenorrheic women.[24] Total protection against pregnancy is achieved by the exclusively breastfeeding woman for a duration of only 10 weeks.

Choice of Contraception

When to Start. Additional contraception is necessary during lactation for most women. That is not to say that full breastfeeding shouldn't be encouraged and that the protection obtained in the first 6 months of breastfeeding shouldn't be emphasized. But after 3 months, the first ovulation can precede the first menstrual bleed.

The Rule of 3's.
In the presence of FULL breastfeeding, a contraceptive method should be used beginning in the *3rd postpartum month*.

With PARTIAL breastfeeding or NO breastfeeding, a contraceptive method should begin during the *3rd postpartum week*.

After the termination of a pregnancy of less than 12 weeks, oral contraception can be started immediately. After a pregnancy of 12 or more weeks, the 3rd postpartum week rule should be followed if the pregnancy is term or near term. The latter delay has been based on a theoretical concern over an increased risk of thrombosis early in the postpartum period. This is probably no longer an issue with low dose oral contraception. *We believe that oral contraception can be initiated immediately after a second trimester abortion or premature delivery.*

The Postpartum Visit. Contraception is usually on the mind of both patient and clinician at the first postpartum visit. A recent pregnancy and a new infant provide strong motivation to consider contraception. Traditonally, the first medical visit after delivery has been scheduled at 6 weeks, a time when good involution of the uterus and healing have occurred. Unfortunately in nonbreastfeeding women, ovulation can occur during the 4th postpartum week. We urge clinicians and patients to start a new tradition: schedule the first postpartum visit during the *3rd week after delivery.* Even breastfeeding women should be evaluated at this time, to consider whether breastfeeding is full and exclusive, or whether an additional contraceptive method is necessary.

Oral Contraception

Oral contraception even in low dose formulations has been demonstrated to diminish the quantity and quality of lactation in postpartum women. Also of concern is the potential hazard of transfer of contraceptive steroids to the infant (a significant amount of the progestational component is secreted into breast milk)[27], however no adverse effects have thus far been identified. Women who use oral contraception have a lower incidence of breastfeeding after the 6th postpartum month, regardless of whether oral contraception is started at the first, second, or third postpartum month.[28–30]

In adequately nourished women, no impairment of infant growth can be detected; presumably compensation is achieved either through supplementary feedings or increased suckling.[31] In an 8-year follow-up study of children breastfed by mothers using oral contraceptives, no effect could be detected on diseases, intelligence, or psychological behavior.[32] This study also found that mothers on birth control pills lactated a significantly shorter period of time than controls, a mean of 3.7 months vs 4.6 months in controls.

Because of the concerns regarding the impact of oral contraceptives on breastfeeding, a useful alternative is to combine the contraceptive effect of lactation with the progestin-only minipill (see Chapter 3). In contrast to the combined oral contraceptive, the progestin-only minipill provides a modest boost to milk production, and women using the minipill breastfeed longer and add supplementary feeding at a later time.[31,33] The combination of lactation and the progestin-only minipill is associated with near total contraceptive efficacy. Because of the positive impact on breastfeeding, the minipill can be started immediately after delivery at or near term.

In patients who prefer the standard low dose combined oral contraceptive, the full breastfeeder should begin during the 3rd postpartum month; all others during the 3rd postpartum week. Starting oral contraception during the 3rd postpartum week safely avoids the hypercoaguable state immediately after delivery.

Long-Acting Methods

Neither Norplant nor Depo-Provera affect breastfeeding.[34,35] These methods are both excellent choices for postpartum contraception. They can be initiated immediately postpartum, but certainly should be utilized no later than the 3rd postpartum week.

Periodic Abstinence

Women skilled in the cervical mucus method can detect evidence of fertile type mucus prior to the first menses in the postpartum period. However, there are many false positive and false negative interpretations.[36] This method cannot be used with a great deal of confidence until regular menses are resumed.

Barrier Methods

Barrier methods, of course, have no impact on breastfeeding, and they are an excellent choice for motivated couples. Lubricated condoms are especially helpful for the vaginal dryness experienced by some breastfeeding women. Spermicides and foam products can also help with the dryness and dyspareunia. It is difficult to fit a diaphragm or cervical cap before healing and involution are complete (about 6 weeks), and it is not advisable to use a sponge, cap, or diaphragm while still bleeding. Therefore spermicides, foam, and condoms should be used in the immediate postpartum period, and use of the sponge, cap, or diaphragm can be started about the 6th postpartum week.

The Postpartum IUD

Modern IUDs can be inserted between 4 and 8 weeks postpartum without an increase in pregnancy rates, expulsion, or removals for bleeding and/or pain.[37]

References

1. Thapa S, Short RV, Potts M, Breastfeeding, birthspacing and child survival, Nature 335:679, 1988.

2. Davidson WD, Durham NC, A brief history of infant feeding, J Pediatrics 43:74, 1953.

3. National Academy of Sciences, *Nutrition During Lactation,* National Academy Press, Washington, D.C., 1991.

4. Ryan AS, Pratt WF, Wysong JL, Lewandowski G, McNally JW, Krieger FW, A comparison of breast-feeding data from the National Surveys of Family Growth and the Ross Laboratories Mothers Surveys, Am J Public Health 81:1049, 1991.

5. Topper YL, Multiple hormone interactions in the development of the mammary gland in vitro, Recent Prog Horm Res 26:287, 1970.

6. Tyson JE, Hwang P, Guyda H, Friesen HG, Studies of prolactin secretion in human pregnancy, Am J Obstet Gynecol 113:14, 1972.

7. Murphy LJ, Murphy LC, Stead B, Sutherland RL, Lazarus L, Modulation of lactogenic receptors by progestins in cultured human breast cancer cells, J Clin Endocrinol Metab 62:280, 1986.

8. Simon WE, Pahnke VG, Holzel F, In vitro modulation of prolactin binding to human mammary carcinoma cells by steroid hormones and prolactin, J Clin Endocrinol Metab 60:1243, 1985.

9. Battin DA, Marrs RP, Fleiss PM, Mishell DR Jr, Effect of suckling on serum prolactin, luteinizing hormone, follicle-stimulating hormone, and estradiol during prolonged lactation, Obstet Gynecol 65:785, 1985.

10. Dawood MY, Khan-Dawood FS, Wahl RS, Fuchs F, Oxytocin release and plasma anterior pituitary and gonadal hormones in women during lactation, J Clin Endocrinol Metab 52:678, 1981.

239

11. Ben-Jonathan N, Dopamine: A prolactin-inhibiting hormone, Endocrin Rev 6:564, 1985.

12. Short RV, Lactation—The central control of reproduction, Ciba Found Symp 45:73, 1976.

13. Tyson JE, Carter JN, Andreassen B, Huth J, Smith B, Nursing mediated prolactin and luteinizing hormone secretion during puerperal lactation, Fertil Steril 30:154, 1978.

14. Sauder SE, Frager M, Case GD, Kelch RP, Marshall JC, Abnormal patterns of pulsatile luteinizing hormone secretion in women with hyperprolactinemia and amenorrhea: Responses to bromocriptine, J Clin Endocrinol Metab 59:941, 1984.

15. Petraglia F, De Leo V, Nappi C, Facchinetti F, Montemagno U, Brambilla F, Genazzani AR, Differences in the opioid control of luteinizing hormone secretion between pathological and iatrogenic hyperprolactinemic states, J Clin Endocrinol Metab 64:508, 1987.

16. Gray RH, Campbell OM, Zacur HA, Labbok MH, MacRae SL, Postpartum return of ovarian activity in nonbreastfeeding women monitored by urinary assays, J Clin Endocrinol Metab 64:645, 1987.

17. Howie PW, McNeilly AS, Houston MJ, et al, Effect of supplementary food on suckling patterns and ovarian activity during lactation, Br Med J 282:757, 1981.

18. Perez A, Vela P, Masnick GS, Potter RG, First ovulation after childbirth: The effect of breastfeeding, Am J Obstet Gynecol 114:1041, 1972.

19. Diaz S, Peralta O, Juez G, Salvatierra AM, Casado ME, Duran E, Croxatto HB, Fertility regulation in nursing women. I. The probablity of conception in full nursing women living in an urban setting, J Biosoc Sci 14:329, 1982.

20. McNeilly AS, Glasier A, Howie PW, Endocrine control of lactational infertility, in Dobbing J, editor, *Maternal Nutrition and Lactational Infertility,* Nevey/Raven Press, New York, 1985, p. 177.

21. Rivera R, Kennedy KI, Ortiz E, Barrera M, Bhiwandiwala PP, Breast-feeding and the return to ovulation in Durango, Mexico, Fertil Steril 49:780, 1988.

22. Lewis PR, Brown JB, Renfree MB, Short RV, The resumption of ovulation and menstruation in a well-nourished population of women breastfeeding for an extended period of time, Fertil Steril 55:529, 1991.

23. Short RV, Lewis PR, Renfree MB, Shaw G, Contraceptive effects of extended lactational amenorrhoea: Beyond the Bellagio Consensus, Lancet 337:715, 1991.

24. Diaz S, Aravena R, Cardenas H, Casado ME, Miranda P, Schiappacasse V, Croxatto HB, Contraceptive efficacy of lactational amenorrhea in urban Chilean women, Contraception 43:335, 1991.

25. Kennedy KI, Rivera R, McNeilly AS, Consensus statement on the use of breastfeeding as a family planning method, Bellagio, Italy, Contraception 39:477, 1989.

26. Gray RH, Campbell OM, Apelo R, Eslami SS, Zacur H, Ramos RM, Gehret JC, Labbok MH, Risk of ovulation during lactation, Lancet 335:25, 1990.

27. Betrabet SS, Shikary ZK, Toddywalla VS, Toddywalla SP, Patel D, Saxena BN, Transfer of norethisterone (NET) and levonorgestrel (LNG) from a single tablet into the infant's circulation through the mother's milk, Contraception 35:517, 1987.

28. Diaz S, Peralta O, Juez G, Herreros C, Casado ME, Salvatierra AM, Miranda P, Durn E, Croxatto HB, Fertility regulation in nursing women: III. Short-term influence of a low-dose combined oral contraceptive upon lactation and infant growth, Contraception 27:1, 1982.

29. Croxatto HB, Diaz S, Peralta O, Juez G, Herreros C, Casado ME, Salvatierra AM, Miranda P, Durn E, Fertility regulation in nursing women: IV. Long-term influence of a low-dose combined oral contraceptive initiated at day 30 postpartum upon lactation and child growth, Contraception 27:13, 1983.

30. Peralta O, Diaz S, Juez G, Herreros C, Casado ME, Salvatierra AM, Miranda P, Durn E, Croxatto HB, Fertility regulation in nursing women: V. Long-term influence of a low-dose combined oral contraceptive initiated at day 90 postpartum upon lactation and infant growth, Contraception 27:27, 1983.

31. WHO Special Programme of Research, Development, and Research Training in Human Reproduction, Task Force on Oral Contraceptives, Effects of hormonal contraceptives on milk volume and infant growth, Contraception 30:505, 1984.

32. Nilsson S, Mellbin T, Hofvander Y, Sundelin C, Valentin J, Nygren KG, Long-term follow-up of children breast-fed by mothers using oral contraceptives, Contraception 34:443, 1986.

33. McCann MF, Moggia AV, Hibbins JE, Potts M, Becker C, The effects of a progestin-only oral contraceptive (levonorgestrel 0.03 mg) on breast-feeding, Contraception 40:635, 1989.

34. Diaz S, Herreros C, Juez G, Casado ME, Salvatierra AM, Miranda P, Peralto O, Croxatto HB, Fertility regulation in nursing women: Influence of Norplant levonorgestrel implants upon lactation and infant growth, Contraception 32:53, 1985.

35. Jimenez J, Ochoa M, Soler MP, Portales P, Long-term follow-up of children breast-fed by mothers receiving depot-medroxyprogesterone acetate, Contraception 30:5232, 1984.

36. Gross BA, Natural family planning indicators of ovulation, Clin Reprod Fertil 5:91, 1987.

37. Mishell DR Jr, Roy S, Copper intrauterine contraceptive device event rates following insertion 4 to 8 weeks post partum, Am J Obstet Gynecol 143:29, 1982.

9

Clinical Guidelines for Contraception at Different Ages

MODERN SOCIETY is coping with two contraceptive problems, each at the opposite end of the reproductive lifespan. In the early years, we are struggling with the high rate of unwanted teenage pregnancies. In the later years, we face a growing demand for reversible contraception as the post World War II baby boom generation ages. It is entirely appropriate, therefore, that we give special attention to these age groups: adolescence and the transition years (ages 35 to menopause).

Contraception for Adolescents

Providing contraception or information about contraception for young people under age 20 is an important obligation for clinicians. More young women become pregnant in the United States than do their contemporaries in other developed parts of the world, and young American women have a higher abortion rate than young European women.[1] More than 50% of the 1.6 million abortions per year in the United States are obtained by women younger than age 25, with the rate peaking at ages 18–19.[2,3]

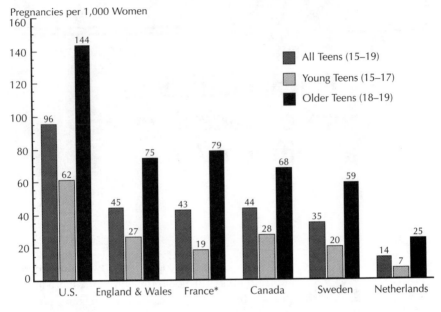

1981 Teenage Pregnancy Rates in the U.S. vs. Other Developed Countries[8]

Pregnancies per 1,000 Women

Legend:
- All Teens (15–19)
- Young Teens (15–17)
- Older Teens (18–19)

*1980 data

There has been a marked increase in teenage sexual activity in the United States during the 1980s, and contrary to common opinion, much of that increase occurred among white and nonpoor adolescents.[4] Within a relatively short period of time after becoming sexually active, 58% of adolescent females have had sex with 2 or more partners (and thus, increase their risk of sexually transmitted diseases [STDs]). By age 17, 50% of teenagers are sexually active.

Characteristics of Teen Pregnancy in the United States[5,6]
1. 3,000 teen pregnancies occur every day.
2. One of every 10 teens aged 15–19 get pregnant.
3. Half of teen pregnancies occur in the first 6 months after first intercourse.
4. 20% of teen pregnancies occur in the first month after first intercourse.
5. Half who give birth do not graduate from high school.

Adolescence is a time for "trying your wings," a time for experimenting and testing. Most of the 25 million teenagers in the United States will make it, but unfortunately for many, the consequences of this time of trying things will be a lasting problem for health and life. Unwanted pregnancy (premature parenthood) and the STDs are the risks of sexual experimentation. Adolescent males should be impressed with the fact that young women carry the burden of unprotected sexual activity: combining unwanted pregnancy with undetected STDs and pelvic inflammatory disease (PID). Screening for chlamydia and culturing for gonorrhea are essential parts of the pelvic examination in sexually active young women.

Teenagers are noted for their sense of invincibility and their risk-taking behavior, both of which denote the inability of immature people to connect present action with future consequences. It is not surprising that adolescents often have sex and do not use contraception. Contraception takes planning and premeditation about having sex. More than half of female teenagers have risked pregnancy by having unprotected intercourse at least once. The onset of fertility following menarche cannot be predicted for individuals; any sexually active teenager is at risk for pregnancy. It is worth emphasizing that there is no evidence that provision of contraception leads to adolescents having sex earlier or more frequently. Repeated studies have documented a constant finding: adolescents seeking contraception usually do so one year *after* initiating sexual activity.

Our objective is to get adolescents to plan sexual involvement, not to just let it happen. The fact that European adolescents use contraception at a rate higher than in the United States argues that we can do better. Unfortunately, secrecy usually surrounds a young person's decision to use contraception; this is associated with a lack of opportunity for reinforcement by family or peers. Access to contraception (physical and psychological) and motivation to use are the keys. Success in achieving our goals requires specific approaches and skills in communicating with adolescents.

245

Topics Teenagers Would Like to Discuss with Physicians [7]

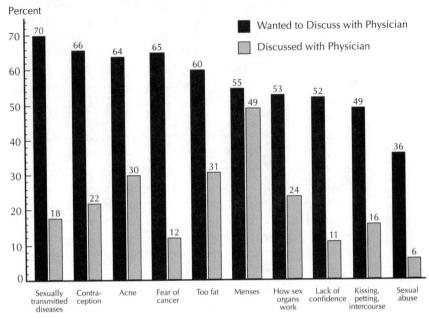

Percent

■ Wanted to Discuss with Physician
▦ Discussed with Physician

	Sexually transmitted diseases	Contraception	Acne	Fear of cancer	Too fat	Menses	How sex organs work	Lack of confidence	Kissing, petting, intercourse	Sexual abuse
Wanted	70	66	64	65	60	55	53	52	49	36
Discussed	18	22	30	12	31	49	24	11	16	6

Communication With Adolescents

Teenagers want to talk about STDs and contraception, but clinicians usually don't bring these subjects up for discussion.[7] Clinicians can be sure that 75% of adolescents will be interested in discussing STDs and contraception by age 15. No matter what brings an adolescent into the office, contraception and compliance are issues that should be addressed.

Our goals are to promote abstinence among teenagers who are not yet ready to cope with responsibility, and to promote behavior to prevent pregnancy and STDs in sexually active adolescents. Building trust is a requirement for a successful interaction between clinician and adolescent. A teenager must be assured that a discussion about sexuality and contraception will be strictly confidential. This must be stated in plain words. One reason European countries are able to provide better contraceptive services to adolescents is the guarantee by law of complete confidentiality (other reasons are dissemination of information via public media and distribution of contraceptives through free or low-cost services).[8] Research confirms that requiring parental notification or consent deters young people from using contraception.

Good compliance requires teenager involvement, not just passive listening. The clinician should frequently interrupt talking by asking questions and seeking opinions. Don't wait until the physical examination to initiate conversation. It is a good practice to see all patients first in an office setting, but this is especially true with adolescents. Give some thought to body language and position. It is helpful to sit next to a patient; avoid the formality (and obstacle) of a desk between clinician and patient. A teenager should be asked about success in school, family life, and behaviors indicative of risk taking.

Don't miss the chance to point out the wisdom of abstinence to a young person who is not yet sexually active, but leave the door open for protection against pregnancy and STDs. Be careful to be nonjudgmental. Sometimes it is hard to keep disapproval over a teenager's activity from showing. A teenager who senses disapproval won't listen to instructions or advice.

A good way to introduce the subject of contraception is to ask an adolescent *when* he or she would like to have children. Then follow with: what plans do you have to avoid getting pregnant until then? Elicit objections, concerns, fears, and address each of them. The clinician must anticipate those concerns and fears which will lead to poor compliance. They must be identified and addressed in advance.

Contraceptive use is a private matter, and therefore, instruction comes from the clinician, not from peers. Be very concrete; demonstrate the use of pill packages, foam aerosols, and sponge and condom application. This seems like oversimplification, but clinicians working with adolescents have found that this approach is both necessary and appreciated by their young patients.

247

Adolescents must be convinced that having sex means you are at risk of becoming pregnant. Adolescents are immersed in conflicting messages about sexuality in our society. A clinician may be the only resource for information and guidance, but clinicians must give the right signals to adolescents and must initiate communication. No matter what the chief complaint, any interaction with an adolescent is an opportunity to discuss sexuality and contraception.

Choice of Method

Oral Contraception. Oral contraception is by far the most popular and most requested method of contraception by teenagers.[9] This is appropriate because oral contraceptives are almost never medically contraindicated in healthy adolescents. The risk of death from oral contraceptive use by adolescents is virtually nil, even for those who smoke heavily. This is a good match; adolescents are at highest risk for unwanted pregnancies and are at lowest risk for complications. Thus, the high efficacy of oral contraception is the best choice for teenagers.

Adolescents certainly don't know the history of oral contraception, but teenagers do have concerns regarding oral contraception, citing most often a fear of cancer, concern with impact on future fertility, and problems with weight gain and acne.[10] It is important to point out the change in dosage and the new safety before addressing these fears.

The cancer issue is a difficult one. We believe it is appropriate to state that there is no definitive evidence demonstrating a link between breast cancer and oral contraception. On the other hand, patients deserve to know of our concern, and the findings regarding long duration of use and the possible increased risk of early, premenopausal breast cancer (Chapter 2). As long as inconsistencies exist in the epidemiologic evidence, the clinician is justified in being optimistic, stating that risk is possible, but it has not been proven. The risk of cervical cancer also continues to be a concern, although confounding factors have been difficult to control. Pap smear surveillance must be emphasized. It is worth pointing out that these data on breast and cervical cancer are derived from older, higher dose pills.

By the time of menarche, growth and reproductive development are essentially complete. There is no evidence that early use of oral contraception has any inhibiting impact on growth or any adverse effects on the reproductive tract. With great confidence, a clinician can tell adolescents that there is no impact on future fertility with the use of oral contraception. Indeed, one can emphasize that oral contraception preserves future fertility by its protection against PID and ectopic pregnancies. While oral contraception protects against PID, it does not protect against contracting STDs, hence the recommendation to combine oral contraception use with barrier methods. *Because it is now relatively common for young women to have changing relationships, a dual approach is recommended, combining the contraceptive efficacy and protection against PID offered by oral contraception with the use of a barrier method (and spermicide) for prevention of viral STDs.*

Repeatedly emphasize to adolescents that studies with low dose oral contraception, even studies in adolescents[11], do not indicate a problem of weight gain and that acne is usually improved. Reassurance about weight gain as it is perceived by the teenager deserves attention at every visit.

Adolescents are especially receptive to hearing about the beneficial impact of oral contraception on menstrual problems: cramps, bleeding, and irregular periods.

Teenage smoking continues to be a big problem, but there is no evidence that young smokers have an increased risk of a cardiovascular event if they use oral contraception.

Adolescents with diabetes mellitus uncomplicated with vascular changes can use oral contraception. Other conditions with which oral contraception is acceptable include cystic fibrosis, sickle cell disease, and seizure disorders controlled by antiepileptic drugs.

Serial monogamy is common among teens, but this often is associated with serial use of contraception. With oral contraception, it is helpful to instruct the adolescent that the minor side effects diminish in frequency with use, and therefore, there is an advantage to staying on the oral contraceptive. It is also good advice to tell teenagers to continue taking oral contraceptives for at least two months after "breaking up" with a boyfriend; by then a new relationship is likely to have begun.

249

Some family planning experts are advocating the elimination of the pelvic examination as a requirement for teenagers to obtain oral contraceptives. One reason the average teenager waits a year after initiating sexual activity before seeking contraception is fear about the pelvic exam. Furthermore, anxiety over the pelvic exam is a barrier to comprehending contraceptive instructions. Thus, delaying the pelvic exam until the 3rd or 6th month may increase access and compliance. This approach requires a completely normal history (an absence of risk factors for STDs) and a limited prescription. Our experience is that teens who were initially wary of the examination will feel more confident with the clinician at the 3 month visit.

Barrier Methods. Teenagers have the highest rates of hospitalization for PID. The following statistics are cited about adolescent, young women:[12]

1. 8–25% of sexually active adolescent females are infected with Chlamydia.
2. 0.4–12% are infected with Neisseria.
3. 15–38% have human papillomavirus infection.
4. 16% of adolescents have abnormal Pap smears.

For these reasons, combined with the AIDS scare, there has been an increase in the use of condoms among adolescents. After oral contraception, in our view, the condom used with a spermicide is the next best choice for adolescents. And this obviously is the only choice for male adolescents. *Indeed, experts in adolescent contraception strongly advocate combining condoms with oral contraception to provide maximum protection against pregnancy and STDs.* Sexually active young women should be examined every 6 months, with Pap smear and STD screening.

The advantage of condoms with spermicide is that neither a prescription nor a consultation with a clinician is required. The problem, then, is achieving sufficient education and motivation without the intervention of clinicians. We believe this is a social problem, not a medical problem, and we are strongly supportive of public education efforts in schools and the media to accomplish this important public and individual health objective.

Many teenagers rely on condoms, and of course their contribution to preventing STDs is important, Condom failures, unfortunately, are about 10 times as high among teenagers as among older, married couples. Don't assume that teenagers know how to use a condom; use a model (a banana works) and demonstrate. Furthermore, young women need to know that they are in charge; they can insist on condom use. Role-playing and practicing a few arguments are helpful.

Diaphragms/cervical caps are not good choices for adolescents. Adolescents are not comfortable with body interventions, and the insertion is too willful an act linked with coitus. Furthermore, this method requires privacy for insertion. Adolescents are discouraged by complicated methods. The diaphragm and cervical cap should be reserved for very motivated and mature young people.

The Intrauterine Device. Traditionally, IUDs have not been recommended for nulliparous women and those who have a high risk of STDs. This eliminates it from consideration for most teenagers. However, we wish to emphasize that age and parity are not the critical factors; the risk for STDs is the most important consideration. The IUD can and should be considered for the older teenager who is married in a stable monogamous relationship and has had a child, and even in the appropriate nulliparous young woman. It is also a good choice in a patient with a chronic illness, such as diabetes mellitus or systemic lupus erythematosus, or in mentally retarded individuals.

Vaginal Contraceptives. The creams, foams, suppositories, and jellies are not ideal for adolescents. They require proper timing and placement for good efficacy. The vaginal sponge is more acceptable. Its efficacy is highest in nulliparous women, and its duration of action lasts 24 hours. Certainly any of these methods is better than nothing.

Norplant and Depo-Provera. Although long-acting contraceptives are an excellent answer to compliance problems, the many minor side effects represent a difficult problem for teenagers. Acne, weight change, and irregular bleeding are more common among Norplant and Depo-Provera users than among oral contraceptive users. In addition the cost and the surgical procedure with Norplant can be major difficulties for adolescents.[13] But there are special candidates for long-acting methods: teens who have failed oral contraception and teens who are mentally retarded or who have chronic illnesses (in which estrogen is contraindicated).

Postcoital Contraception. Because adolescents often have unplanned sexual intercourse, access to emergency postcoital contraception is important. (Chapter 3) The failure rate is approximately 1%. Treatment should be initiated as soon after exposure as possible, but no later than 72 hours. Side effects reflect the high doses used: nausea, vomiting, headache, dizziness. We recommend the 50 μg estrogen combination pill as follows:[14]

Ovral, 4 tablets (2 given 12 hours apart).

Adolescent Compliance

Knowing that contraception is available is not enough to prevent adolescent pregnancy. Adolescents have higher failure rates with all methods. Adolescent compliance with oral contraception has been particularly well-studied.[15,16] Factors associated with good compliance include: older age, suburban residence, health care in a private practice, payment status, prior use of contraception, mother's *unawareness* of oral contraception, married parents, older boyfriend, and satisfaction with pill use. Good compliance is also associated with educational goals and an absence of side effects. Inner city teens express more concern with side effects and safety, while suburban patients are more worried about weight gain and the effect of smoking. Surprisingly, in a study of 214 patients, only 11 reported reading the written instruction sheets which were provided.[15]

These studies indicate the importance of verbal instructions and the need to allow for questions. Long-term compliance is associated with an adolescent's career goals; it is worth bringing this up in conversation. Because adolescents tend to switch methods, all methods should be discussed with adolescents at each visit. Studies demonstrate that the extra time and effort required to meet the needs of adolescents result in improved contraceptive use and lower pregnancy rates.[17]

Keys to Improving Adolescent Compliance
1. Establish and maintain confidentiality to build trust.
2. Do not lecture; make the patient visit a conversation.
3. Identify and address fears and concerns in advance.
4. Emphasize benefits.
5. Emphasize that minor side effects with oral contraception diminish with use.
6. Give instructions for managing side effects and what to do if pills are missed.
7. Demonstrate use of the package and pill taking as well as condom application.
8. Incorporate pill taking into a patient's daily routine.
9. Don't let patients run out of pills.
10. Request that you be called before oral contraception is discontinued.
11. Identify and educate office personnel to interact with adolescents.
12. Frequent visits (every 3 months the first year), short waiting time, convenient hours.

Contraception for Older Women

The years from age 35 to menopause can be referred to as the transition years. During this period of time, there are several medical needs which must be addressed: the need for contraception, the management of persistent anovulation, and finally, menopausal and postmenopausal hormone replacement therapy.

At approximately 40 years of age, the frequency of ovulation decreases. This initiates a period of waning ovarian function called the climacteric, which will last several years, carrying a woman through decreased fertility and menopause, to the postmenopausal years. Prior to menopause, the remaining follicles perform less well. During this period, women who are having regular periods can have lower estradiol levels and higher levels of FSH, and the cycle begins to change, mainly because of a shortening of the follicular phase.

As cycles become irregular, vaginal bleeding occurs at the end of an inadequate luteal phase or after a peak of estradiol without subsequent ovulation and corpus luteum formation. Eventually, many women live through a period of oligoanovulation. Occasionally corpus luteum formation and function occur, and therefore, the oligoanovulatory woman is not totally safe from the threat of an unplanned and unexpected pregnancy.

In Chapter 1, we pointed out that the need for reversible contraception by women over 30 is increasing. More and more couples are deferring pregnancy until later in life, and therefore, the use of sterilization will decline. For the next 20 years, as the post World War II baby boom generation ages, there will be an unprecedented number of women in the later child-bearing years.

253

The Intrauterine Device

The IUD is a good reversible contraceptive choice for older women. An older woman is more likely to be mutually monogamous and less likely to develop PID, and for those women who have already had their children, concern with fertility and problems with cramping and bleeding are both lesser issues. If protection from STDs is not a concern, insertion of a copper IUD can provide very effective contraception until the menopause without the need to do anything other than check the string occasionally. On the other hand, because alterations of bleeding patterns become more common in this age group, it may be necessary to remove an IUD.

Barrier Methods

Some women use barrier methods throughout their reproductive years, but most change to easier, more effective methods as their sexual lives become more stable, their risk of STDs decreases accordingly, and they need contraception for avoiding rather than spacing pregnancies. Some women begin new relationships as they age and may require reminding about the risks of STDs and the need to use condoms with new partners whose sexual and drug use histories are unknown. Perimenopausal women whose earlier use of contraception was not directed at avoiding HIV infection may need to learn how and with whom to use condoms.

Long-Acting Contraception

The long-acting methods of hormonal contraception (Norplant and Depo-Provera) deserve consideration in those situations where combination estrogen-progestin is unacceptable due to health problems (where estrogen is contraindicated), or where oral contraception has already proved to be unsuccessful. Older women, as they approach the menopause, may be more comfortable with the irregular bleeding or amenorrhea associated with these methods. Hormone replacement treatment can be initiated if menopausal symptoms develop, or when annual measurement of the FSH level (beginning at age 50) indicates a rise above 30 mIU/ml.

Oral Contraception for the Transitional Years

Fortunately clinicians and patients have recognized that low dose oral contraception is very safe for healthy, nonsmoking older women. However, their use is still not sufficient to meet the need. Among women using contraception in 1988, only 5% of women aged 35–44 used oral contraception and only 3% aged 40–44, compared to 68% aged 20–24.[18] Besides fulfilling a need, we would argue that this population of women has a series of benefits to be derived from oral contraception that tilts the risk/benefit ratio to the positive side. The following benefits are especially pertinent for older women:

254

Effective contraception.
- less need for therapeutic abortion.
- less need for surgical sterilization.

Less endometrial cancer.
Less ovarian cancer.
Less benign breast disease.
Fewer ovarian cysts.
Fewer uterine fibroids.
Fewer ectopic pregnancies.
More regular menses.
- less flow.
- less dysmenorrhea.
- less anemia.

Less salpingitis.
Less rheumatoid arthritis.
Increased bone density.
Probably less endometriosis.
Possibly protection against atherosclerosis.

The most up-to-date conclusion now indicates that the risk of dying from circulatory diseases is confined to smokers over the age of 35 who use oral contraception, and that conclusion is based upon data from women using higher dose pills (Chapter 2). Non-smoking, healthy women over 35 can expect no adverse impact from low dose oral contraception.

Presently there is no reason why low dose oral contraception cannot be utilized by appropriate patients until menopause. Menopause occurs in American women between the ages of 48 and 55, with the median age being approximately 50. Because the age of menopause occurs over such a relatively large age range, it is difficult to know when it is safe to change from oral contraception to a hormonal replacement program. And it should be emphasized that this change is important because the estrogen dose in even the lowest contraceptive formulations available is at least four times greater than what is needed for postmenopausal treatment. However, even this dose of estrogen has an insignificant impact on the coagulation system.[19,20]

The therapeutic principle remains to utilize the formulation which gives effective contraception and the greatest margin of safety. Because we now appreciate the dose-response relationship between the steroid components and side effects, it makes sense to use the lowest doses that are still effective. For this reason products with less

255

than 30 μg of estrogen might be especially useful for older women.

Over the years, the debate over the cause of circulatory complications attributed to oral contraception turned from thrombosis to atherosclerosis. Today, belief is firmly back in the camp of thrombosis. A significant reason is the failure to detect any lingering risk of cardiovascular disease in former pill users. Most noteworthy is the Nurses' Health Study.[21] Now that the nurses initially enrolled in this follow-up study have aged sufficiently, we have statistically and clinically significant data from women who have reached the age of major risk for cardiovascular disease. Even the use of higher-dose oral contraceptives is not associated with a subsequent increased risk of coronary heart disease and stroke. The fact that an increased risk of cardiovascular disease is limited to current use (of higher dose pills) is a very strong indicator that the mechanism is a short-term acute mechanism, specifically thrombosis, an estrogen-related effect. Therefore, our return to the belief that cardiovascular disease is linked to thrombosis makes the role, and the dose, of estrogen very important.

An European product containing 20 μg ethinyl estradiol and 150 μg desogestrel has been demonstrated in a multicenter study of 434 women over age 30 to have the same efficacy and side effects as pills containing 30 and 35 μg of estrogen. [22,23] In a randomized study, this formulation was associated with the virtual elimination of any effects on coagulation factors.[20]

It seems to us that the time is right for the lowest estrogen dose products for older women. While it is true that the implied safety of the lowest estrogen dose remains to be documented by epidemiologic studies, it seems clinically prudent to maximize the safety margin in this older age group of women. Although there may be some increase in breakthrough bleeding, we believe that older women who understand the increased safety implicit in the lowest estrogen dose are more willing to endure breakthrough bleeding and maintain compliance. Clinicians need not be worried that irregular bleeding represents endometrial cancer because the progestational impact will protect the endometrium. With avoidance of risk factors and use of lowest dose pills, health risks are probably negligible for healthy, nonsmoking women. For healthy nonsmoking women, no specific laboratory screening is necessary beyond that which is usually incorporated in a program of preventive health care.

We should also mention the progestin-only minipill (Chapter 3). Because of reduced fecundity, the minipill achieves near total efficacy in women over age 40. Therefore, the progestin-only minipill is a good choice for older women, and especially for those women in whom estrogen is contraindicated. Older women are more accepting of irregular menstrual bleeding when they understand its mechanism, and thus, are more accepting of the progestin-only minipill.

When to Change from Oral Contraception to HRT. One approach to establish the onset of the postmenopausal years is to measure the FSH level, beginning at age 50, on an annual basis, being careful to obtain the blood sample on day 6 or 7 of the pill-free week. By then, the steroid levels will have declined sufficiently to allow FSH to rise. When FSH is greater than 30 mIU/ml, it is time to change to a hormone replacement program. Some clinicians are comfortable allowing patients to enter their mid-fifties on low dose oral contraception, and then empirically switching to a hormone replacement regimen.

Anovulation and Bleeding. Throughout the transitional period of life there is a significant incidence of dysfunctional uterine bleeding due to anovulation. While the clinician is usually alerted to this problem because of irregular bleeding, clinician and patient often fail to diagnose anovulation when bleeding is not abnormal in schedule, flow, or duration. As a woman approaches menopause, a more aggressive attempt to document ovulation is warranted. A serum progesterone level measured approximately one week before menses is simple enough to obtain and worth the cost. The prompt diagnosis of anovulation (serum progesterone less than 300 ng/dl) will lead to appropriate therapeutic management which will have a significant impact on the risk of endometrial cancer.

In an anovulatory woman with proliferative or hyperplastic endometrium (unaccompanied by atypia), periodic oral progestin therapy is mandatory, such as 10 mg medroxyprogesterone acetate given daily the first 10 days of each month. If hyperplasia is already present, follow-up aspiration office curettage after 3–4 months is required. If progestin treatment is ineffective and histological regression is not observed, more aggressive treatment is warranted.

Monthly progestin treatment should be continued until withdrawal bleeding ceases or menopausal symptoms are experienced. These are reliable signs (in effect, a bioassay) indicating the onset of estrogen deprivation and the need for the addition of estrogen in a postmenopausal hormone replacement program.

If contraception is desired, the clinician and patient should seriously consider the use of oral contraception. The anovulatory woman cannot be guaranteed that spontaneous ovulation and pregnancy will not occur. The use of a low dose oral contraceptive will at the same time provide contraception and prophylaxis against irregular, heavy anovulatory bleeding and the risk of endometrial hyperplasia and neoplasia.

Clinicians have been made so wary of providing oral contraceptives to older women that a traditional hormone replacement regimen is often utilized to treat a woman with the kind of irregular cycles usually experienced in the transitional years. This addition of exogenous estrogen when a woman is not amenorrheic or experiencing menopausal symptoms is inappropriate, and even risky (exposing the endometrium to excessively high levels of estrogen). The appropriate response is to regulate anovulatory cycles with monthly progestational treatment or to utilize low dose oral contraception.

Conclusion. Preventive health care for women is especially important during the transition years. The issues of preventive health care are familiar ones. They include contraception, cessation of smoking, prevention of heart disease and osteoporosis, maintenance of mental well-being (including sexuality), and cancer screening. Management of the transition years should be significantly oriented to preventive health care, and the use of low dose oral contraception can now legitimately be viewed as a component of preventive health care. A discussion of the noncontraceptive health benefits of low dose oral contraception is especially important with patients in their transition years. This group of women appreciates and understands decisions made with the risk-benefit ratio in mind.

References

1. Westoff CF, Unintended pregnancy in America and abroad, Fam Plann Perspect 20:254, 1988.

2. Henshaw SK, Van Vort J, Teenage abortion, birth and pregnancy statistics: An update, Fam Plann Perspect 21:85, 1989.

3. Henshaw SK, Van Vort J, Abortion services in the United States, 1987 and 1988, Fam Plann Perspect 22:102, 1990.

4. Forrest JD, Singh S, The sexual and reproductive behavior of American women, 1982–1988, Fam Plann Perspect 22:206, 1990.

5. Zabin LS, Kanatner JF, Zelnick M, The risk of adolescent pregnancy in the first months of intercourse, Fam Plann Perspect 11:215, 1979,

6. Trussell J, Teenage pregnancy in the United States, Fam Plann Perspect 20:262, 1989.

7. Malus M, LaChance PA, Lamy L, Macaulay A, Vanasse M, Priorities in adolescent health care: The teenager's viewpoint, J Fam Pract 25:159, 1987.

8. Jones EF, Forrest JD, Goldman N, et al, Teenage pregnancy in developed countries: Determinants and policy implications, Fam Plann Perspect 17:53, 1985.

9. Jay MS, Bridges CE, Gottlieb A, et al, Adolescent contraception, Adolesc Pediatr Gynecol 1:83, 1988.

10. Jay MS, DuRant RH, Litt IF, Female adolescents' compliance with contraceptive regimens, Ped Clinics N Am 36:731, 1989.

11. Carpenter S, Neinstein LS, Weight gain in adolescent and young adult oral contraceptive users, J Adolesc Health Care 7:342, 1986.

12. Werner MJ, Biro FM, Contraception and sexually transmitted diseases in adolescent females, Adolesc Pediatr Gynecol 3:127, 1990.

259

13. Darney PD, Klaisle CM, Tanner S, Alvarado AM, Sustained-release contraceptives, Curr Probl Obstet Gynecol Fertil 13:95, 1990.

14. Bagshaw SN, Edwards D, Tucker AK, Ethinyl estradiol and d-norgestrel is an effective emergency postcoital contraceptive: A report of its use in 1200 patients in a family planning clinic, Aust N Z J Obstet Gynaecol 28:137, 1988.

15. Emans SJ, Grace E, Woods ER, Smith DE, Klein K, Merola J, Adolescents' compliance with the use of oral contraceptives, JAMA 257:3377, 1987,

16. DuRant RH, Jay S, Linder CW, et al, The influence of psycho-social factors on adolescent compliance with oral contraceptives, J Adolesc Health, in press.

17. Winter L, Breckenmaker LC, Tailoring family planning services to the special needs of adolescents, Fam Plann Perspect 23:24, 1991.

18. Mosher WD, Contraceptive practice in the United States, 1982–1988, Fam Plann Perspect 22:198, 1990.

19. Gordon MG, Williams SR, Frenchek B, Maxur CH, Speroff L, Dose-dependent effects of postmenopausal estrogen/progestin on antithrombin III and factor XII, J Lab Clin Med 111:52, 1988.

20. Mellis GB, Fruzzetti F, Nicoletti I, Ricci C, Lammers P, Atsma WJ, Fioretti P, A comparative study on the effects of a monophasic pill containing desogestrel plus 20 µg ethinylestradiol, a triphasic combination containing levonorgestel and a monophasic combination containing gestodene on coagulatory factors, Contraception 43:23, 1991.

21. Stampfer MJ, Willett WC, Colditz GA, Speizer FE, Hennekens CH, Past use of oral contraceptives and cardiovascular disease: A meta-analysis in the context of the Nurses' Health Study, Am J Obstet Gynecol 163:285, 1990.

22. Fioretti P, Fruzzetti F, Navalesi R, Ricci C, Moccoli R, Cerri FM, Orlandi MC, Melis GB, Clinical and metabolic study of a new pill containing 20 mcg ethinylestradiol plus 0.150 mg desogestrel, Contraception 35:229, 1987.

23. Steffensen K, Evaluation of an oral contraceptive containing 0.150 desogestrel and 0.020 mg ethinylestradiol in women aged 30 years or older, Acta Obstet Gynecol Scand Suppl 144:23, 1987.

10

Sterilization and Abortion

ONTRACEPTIVE METHODS today are very safe and effective, however, we remain decades away from a perfect method of contraception for either women or men. Because reversible contraceptive methods are not perfect, more than a third of American couples use sterilization instead. In addition, abortion is utilized more often in the U.S. than in most of the rest of the world (see Chapter 1).

Over the past 20 years, nearly a million Americans each year have undergone a sterilization operation, and recently, more women than men. By 1988, 24% of reproductive aged women relied on contraceptive sterilization, 17% by tubal occlusion, and 7% depended upon their partners' vasectomies.[1,2]

Americans use sterilization for contraceptive purposes more than any other country, in our view, because the intrauterine device (the IUD) and oral contraception have a worse reputation here than in the rest of the world. Publicity about side effects and litigation have frightened prospective users, and it is little wonder that Americans turn to sterilization more often and at an earlier age, and, we believe, before they really want to. A significant increase in both female and male sterilization occurred between 1973 and 1988, a period during which the use of IUDs declined and the use of oral contraception decreased substantially, although since the late 1980s, oral contraception has regained some of its popularity.

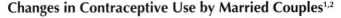

Changes in Contraceptive Use by Married Couples[1,2]

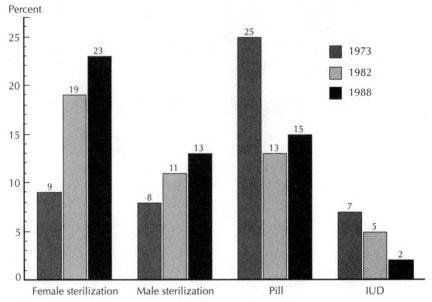

Percent

Legend:
- 1973
- 1982
- 1988

Female sterilization: 9, 19, 23
Male sterilization: 8, 11, 13
Pill: 25, 13, 15
IUD: 7, 5, 2

Since 1980, approximately 1.6 million abortions are performed in the U.S. every year.[3] American teenagers are especially dependent upon abortion compared to their European counterparts who are better educated about sex and use contraception more often and more effectively. In addition, from ages 20–34, American women have the highest proportion of pregnancies aborted compared to other countries, indicating an unappreciated, but real, problem of unintended pregnancy occuring beyond the teenage years. The lack of perfect contraception and imperfect use of contraception will keep abortion with us.

Sterilization and abortion are such common surgical procedures that all clinicians who provide care for women, even those who do not perform these operations, will be involved with questions related to patient's decisions and problems. It is not our intent to teach surgical procedures, but rather to address concerns and questions regarding sterilization and abortion.

Sterilization

James Blundell proposed in 1823, in lectures at Guy's Hospital in London, that tubectomy ought to be performed at cesarean section to avoid the need for repeat sections.[4] He also proposed a technique for sterilization which he later described so precisely that he must actually have performed the operation, although he never wrote about it. The first report was published in 1881 by Samuel Lungren of Toledo, Ohio, who ligated the tubes at the time of cesarean section, as Blundell had suggested 58 years earlier.[5] The Madlener procedure was devised in Germany in 1910 and reported in 1919. Because of many failures, the Madlener technique was supplanted in the U.S. by the method of Ralph Pomeroy, a prominent physician in Brooklyn, New York. This method, still popular today, was not described to the medical profession by Pomeroy's associates until 1929, 4 years after Pomeroy's death. Frederick Irving of the Harvard Medical School described his technique in 1924, and the Uchida method was not reported until 1946.

Few sterilizations were performed until the 1930s when "family planning" was first suggested as an indication by Baird in Aberdeen. He required women to be over 40 and to have had 8 or more children. Mathematical formulas of this kind persisted through the 1960s.

Laparoscopic methods were introduced in the early 1970s. The annual number of vasectomies began to decline, and the number of tubal occlusion operations increased rapidly. By 1973, more sterilization operations were performed for women than for men. This is accurately attributed to dramatic decreases in costs, hospital time, and pain due to the introduction of laparoscopy and minilaparotomy methods. The use of laparoscopy for tubal occlusion increased from only 0.6% of sterilizations in 1970 to more than 35% by 1975.[6] Since 1975, minilaparotomy, a technique popular in the less developed world, has been increasingly performed in the U.S. These methods have allowed women to undergo sterilization operations at times other than immediately after childbirth or during major surgery.

The Pomeroy

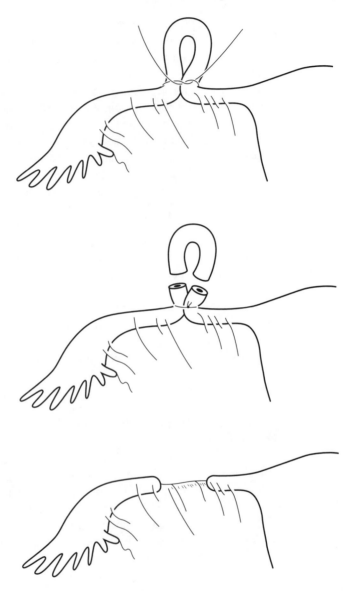

The Irving

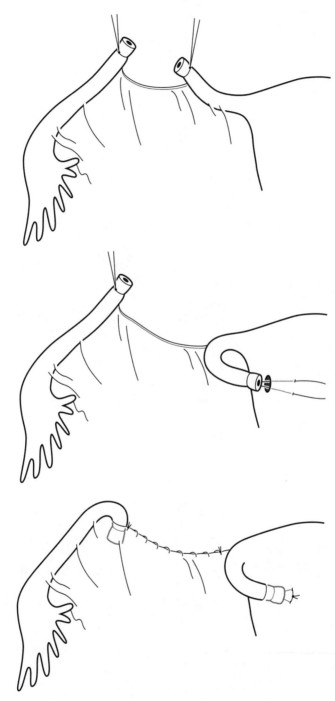

The Uchida

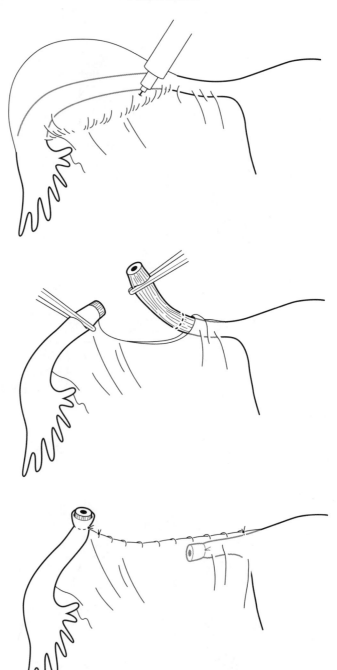

Laparoscopy and minilaparotomy have led to a profound change in the convenience and cost of sterilization operations for women. In 1970, the average woman stayed in the hospital 6.5 days for a tubal sterilization. By 1975, this had declined to 3 days, and today, women rarely remain in the hospital overnight. The shorter length of stay achieved from 1970 to 1975 represented a savings of more than 200 million dollars yearly in health care costs and a tremendous increase in convenience for women eager to return to work and their families.[7] Unlike some advances in technology, laparoscopy and minilaparotomy sterilization are technical innovations which have resulted in large savings in medical care costs. New methods are currently being investigated employing hysteroscopy and transcervical application of substances to obstruct the fallopian tubes.

The great majority of sterilization procedures are accomplished in hospitals by physicians in private practice, but a rapidly increasing proportion are performed outside of hospitals in ambulatory surgical settings, including physician's offices. In either hospital or outpatient settings, female sterilization is a very safe operation. Deaths specifically attributed to sterilization now account for a fatality rate of only 1.5 per 100,000 procedures, a mortality rate that is lower than that for childbearing (about 10 per 100,000 births in the U.S.).[8] When the risk of pregnancy from contraceptive method failure is taken into account, sterilization is the safest of all contraceptive methods.

Vasectomy has long been more popular in the U.S. than anywhere else in the world, but why don't more men use it? One explanation is that women have chosen laparoscopic sterilization in increasing numbers. Another is that men have been frightened by reports, often from animal data, of associations with autoimmune diseases, atherosclerosis, and most recently, prostatic cancer. Large epidemiologic studies have failed to confirm any of these associations. When patients consider sterilization, we can assure them that vasectomy has not been demonstrated to have any harmful effects on men's health.[9] In addition, vasectomy is less expensive, morbidity is less, and mortality is essentially zero.

Efficacy of Sterilization

Laparoscopic and minilaparotomy sterilization are not only convenient, they are almost as effective at preventing pregnancy as were the older, more complex operations. Vasectomy is also highly effective once the supply of remaining sperm in the vas deferens is exhausted. After 6 weeks or 15 ejaculations, essentially all men are sterile.

Failure Rates During the First Year, United States [10]

| Method | Percent of Women with Pregnancy | |
	Lowest Expected	Typical
Female sterilization	0.2%	0.4%
Male sterilization	0.1%	0.15%

Besides the specific operation employed, the skill of the operator and characteristics of the patient make important contributions to the efficacy of female sterilization. Up to 50% of failures are due to technical errors. The methods employing complicated equipment, such as spring-loaded clips and silastic rings, fail for technical reasons more commonly than did simpler procedures such as the Pomeroy tubal ligation.[11] Minilaparotomy failures, therefore, occur much less frequently due to technical errors.

It is hardly surprising that more complicated techniques of tubal occlusion have higher technical failure rates. What is surprising is the finding that characteristics of the patient influence the likelihood of failure even when technical problems are considered. In a careful study of this issue, two patient characteristics, age and lactation, demonstrated a significant impact.[12] Patients younger than 35 years were 1.7 times more likely to become pregnant, and women who were not breastfeeding following sterilization were 5 times more likely to become pregnant. These findings probably reflect the greater fecundity of younger women and the contraceptive contribution of lactation.

Significant numbers of pregnancies following tubal occlusion are present before the procedure. For this reason, some clinicians routinely perform a uterine evacuation or curettage prior to tubal occlusion. It seems more reasonable (and cost effective) to exclude pregnancy by careful history taking, physical examination, and an appropriate pregnancy test prior to the sterilization procedure.[13]

Because method, operator, and patient characteristics all influence sterilization failures, it is difficult to predict which individual will experience a pregnancy after undergoing a tubal occlusion. Therefore, during the course of counseling, all patients should be made aware of the possibility of failure as well as the intent to cause permanent, irreversible sterility. It is important to avoid giving patients the impression that the tubal occlusion procedure is foolproof or guaranteed. Individual clinicians must be cautious judging their own success in accomplishing sterilization, because failure is infrequent and many patients who become pregnant following sterilization never reveal the failure to the original surgeon.

Ectopic pregnancies can occur following tubal occlusion, and the incidence is much higher with some types of tubal occlusion. Bipolar tubal coagulation is more likely to result in ectopic pregnancy than is mechanical occlusion.[11,14] The probable explanation is that microscopic fistulae in the coagulated segment connecting to the peritoneal cavity permit sperm to reach the ovum. Ectopic pregnancies following tubal ligation are more likely to occur 2 or more years after sterilization, rather than immediately after. In the first year after sterilization, about 6% of pregnancies will be ectopic, but the majority of pregnancies which occur 2–3 years after occlusion will be ectopic.[15] The rate of intrauterine pregnancies decreases with time, but ectopic rates remain constant. Overall, however, the risk of an ectopic pregnancy in sterilized women is lower than if they had not been sterilized.

Vaginal procedures have higher failure rates than laparoscopy or minilaparotomy, but the principal disadvantage is higher infection rates. Intraperitoneal infection is a rare complication of minilap or laparoscopic techniques, but in vaginal procedures, abscess formation approaches 1%.[16] This risk can be reduced by the use of prophylactic antibiotics administered intraoperatively, but open laparoscopy is usually easier and safer than vaginal sterilization even in obese women.

Female Sterilization Techniques

Because laparoscopy permits direct visualization and manipulation of the abdominal and pelvic organs with minimal abdominal disruption, it offers many advantages. Hospitalization is not required; most patients return home within a few hours, and the majority return to full activity within 24 hours. Discomfort is minimal, the incision scars are barely visible, and sexual activity need not be restricted. In addition, the surgeon has an opportunity to inspect the pelvic and abdominal organs for abnormalities. The disadvantages of laparoscopic sterilization include the cost, the expensive, fragile equipment, the special training required, and the risks of inadvertent bowel or vessel injury.

Laparoscopic sterilization can be achieved with any of these methods:

1. Occlusion and partial resection by unipolar electrosurgery.
2. Occlusion and transection by unipolar electrosurgery.
3. Occlusion by bipolar electrocoagulation.
4. Occlusion by mechanical means (clips or silastic rings).

All of these methods can use an operating laparoscope alone, or the diagnostic laparoscope with operating instruments passed through a second trocar, or both the operating laparoscope and secondary puncture equipment. All can be employed using the "open" laparoscopic technique in which the laparoscopic instrument is placed into the abdominal cavity under direct vision to avoid the risk of bowel or blood vessel puncture on blind entry. Patient acceptance and recovery are approximately the same with all methods.

Early reports of laparoscopic sterilization revealed that electrocoagulation was not without hazard. Complications were attributed to defective coagulation equipment or inadvertent coagulation of the bowel.[18] These complications can be reduced by establishing a consistent operating protocol and an education program for all operating room personnel, particularly with respect to electrosurgical principles and techniques.

Failure Rates, United States [17]

Pomeroy tubal ligation	4 per 1,000
The Irving tubal ligation	nil
The Uchida tubal ligation	nil
Unipolar electrocoagulation	1 per 1,000
Bipolar electrocoagulation	4 per 1,000
The Hulka-Clemens spring clip	2 per 1,000
The Filshie clip	1 per 1,000
The silastic (Falope or Yoon) ring	4 per 1,000

Tubal Occlusion by Electrosurgical Methods. If electrons from an electrosurgical generator are concentrated in one location, heat within the tissue increases sharply and desiccates the tissue until resistance is so high that no more current can pass. Unipolar methods of sterilization create a dense area of current under the grasping forceps of the unipolar electrode. In order to complete the circuit, however, these electrons must spread through the body and be returned to the generator via a return electrode (the ground plate) which has a broad surface to minimize the density of the current to avoid burns as the electrons leave the body. "Unipolar" refers to the method which requires the patient ground plate.

With the unipolar method, if tissue resistance is high and the electrical pressure (voltage) relatively low, current may cease to flow or may search out alternate pathways with lower resistance. When the voltage is increased, the electrons have more "push" to find another pathway, therefore the surgeon must use the lowest possible voltage necessary to completely coagulate. The return electrode (the ground plate) must be in good contact with the patient.

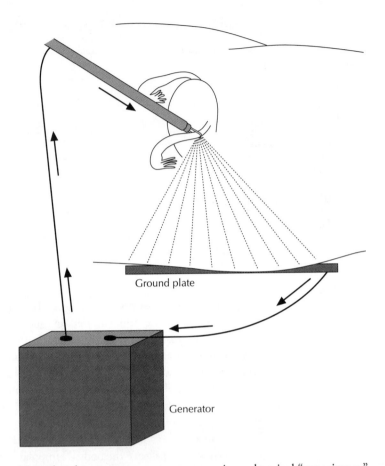

Ground plate

Generator

Unipolar electrosurgery can create a unique electrical "capacitance" problem when an operating laparoscope is used with unipolar forceps. A capacitor is any device that can hold an electric charge, and can exist wherever an insulated material separates two conductors that have different potentials. This property of capacitance explains some of the inadvertent bowel burns that have occurred with laparoscopic sterilization. The operating laparoscope is a hollow metal tube surrounding an active electrode, the forceps used to grasp and coagulate the tubes. When current passes through the active electrode, the laparoscope itself becomes a capacitor. Up to 70% of the current passed through the active electrode can be induced into the laparoscope. Should bowel or other structures touch a laparoscope which is insulated from the abdominal incision (for example, by a fiberglass cannula), the stored electrons will be discharged at high density directly into the vital organ. This potential hazard is eliminated by using a metal trocar sleeve rather than a nonconductive sleeve like fiberglass. Because there is little pressure behind the electrons from a low-voltage generator, not enough heat is generated to burn the skin as the capacitance current leaks out into the patient's body through the sleeve. Even if the active electrode comes in direct contact with the laparoscope, as when a two-incision technique is employed, the current will leak harmlessly through the metal trocar sleeve. The risk of inadvertent coagulation of bowel or other organs cannot be completely eliminated because all body surfaces offer a path back to the ground plate.

The unipolar electrosurgical technique is straightforward. The isthmic portion of the fallopian tube is grasped, elevated away from the surrounding structures and the electrical energy applied until the tissue blanches, swells, and then collapses. The tube is then grasped, moving toward the uterus, recoagulated, and the steps repeated until 2–3 cm of tube have been coagulated. Some surgeons advise against cornual coagulation for fear it may increase the risk of ectopic pregnancy due to fistula formation.

The coagulation and transection technique is performed in a similar fashion with the same instruments. In order to transect the tube, however, an instrument designed to cut tissue must be utilized. The transection of tissue increases the risk of possible bleeding and does not, by itself, reduce the failure rate over coagulation alone. The specimens obtained by this method are usually coagulated beyond microscopic recognition, and therefore, will not provide pathological evidence of successful sterilization.

The bipolar method of sterilization eliminates the ground plate required for unipolar electrosurgery and employs a specially designed forceps. One jaw of the forceps is the active electrode and the other jaw is the ground electrode. Current density is great at the point of forceps contact with tissue, and the use of a low voltage, high-frequency current prevents the spread of electrons. By eliminating the return electrode, the chance of an aberrant pathway through bowel or other structures is greatly reduced. There is, however, a disadvantage with this technique. Since electron spread is decreased, more applications of the grasping forceps are necessary to coagulate the same length of tube than with unipolar coagulation. As desiccation occurs at the point of high current density, tissue resistance increases, and the coagulated area eventually provides resistance to flow of the low-voltage current. Should the resistance increase beyond the voltage's capability to push electrons through the tissue, incomplete coagulation of the endosalpinx can result.[19] In addition, the desiccated tissue can adhere to the bipolar forceps, making it difficult to remove from the surface of the tube.

The bipolar method can be used with either a single incision operating laparoscope or with dual incision instruments. The forceps are, however, more delicate than unipolar equipment and must be kept meticulously clean. Damage to the instruments can alter the ability to coagulate, and inadequate or incomplete electrocoagulation is the main cause of failure.

Bipolar cautery is safer than unipolar cautery with regard to burns of abdominal organs, but most studies indicate higher failure rates. Although the bipolar forceps will not burn tissues that are not actually grasped, care must be taken to avoid coagulating structures adherent to the tubes. For example, the ureter can be damaged when the tube is adherent to the pelvic side wall.

Tubal Occlusion with Clips and Rings. Female sterilization by mechanical occlusion eliminates the safety concerns with electrosurgery. However, mechanical devices are subject to flaws in material, defects in manufacturing, and errors in design; all of which can alter efficacy. Three mechanical devices have been widely used and have low failure rates with long-term follow-up: the Hulka-Clemen's (spring) clip, the Filshie Clip, and the silastic (Falope or Yoon) ring. Each of the three requires an understanding of its mechanical function, a working knowledge of the intricate applicator necessary to apply the device, meticulous attention to maintenance of the applicators, and skillful tubal placement.

Hulka-Clemens Spring Clip. The spring clip consists of two plastic jaws made of Lexan, hinged by a small metal pin 2 mm from one end. Each jaw has teeth on the opposed surface, and a stainless steel spring is pushed over the jaws to hold them closed over the tube. A special laparoscope for one incision application is most commonly employed, although the spring clip can also be used in a two incision procedure. The spring clip destroys 3 mm of tube and has one year pregnancy rates of 2 per 1,000 women.[11]

276

The Hulka-Clemens Spring Clip

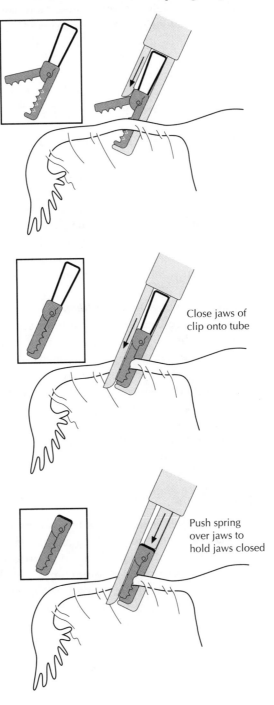

Close jaws of
clip onto tube

Push spring
over jaws to
hold jaws closed

Complications unique to spring clip sterilization result from mechanical difficulties. Should the clip be dislodged or dropped into the abdomen during the procedure, it should be retrieved. Usually it can be removed laparoscopically, but sometimes laparotomy is necessary. Should incomplete occlusion or incorrect alignment of the clip occur, a second clip can be applied without hazard. This clip offers a good chance for reanastomosis, better than electrosurgical methods which destroy more tube.

Filshie Clip. The Filshie clip is made of titanium lined with silicone rubber. The hinged clip is locked over the tube using a special applicator through a second incision or operating laparoscope. The rubber lining of the clip expands on compression to keep the tube blocked. Only 4 mm of the tube is destroyed. Failure rates with the newest model approximate 1 per 1,000 women. Because the Filshie clip is longer, it is reported to occlude dilated tubes more readily than does the spring clip. Both the spring clip and the Filshie clip provide good chances for tubal reanastomosis.

Silastic (Falope or Yoon) Ring. The nonreactive silastic rubber band has an elastic memory of 100% if stretched to no more than 6 mm for a brief time (a few minutes at most). A special applicator, 6 mm in diameter, can be placed through a second cannula, or through a standard offset operating laparoscope. The applicator is designed to grasp a knuckle of tube and release the silastic band onto a 2.5 cm loop of tube. The avascular loop of tube can be resected with biopsy forceps to provide a pathology specimen, but this is rarely done (it does not increase efficacy). Ten to 15% of patients experience severe postoperative pelvic cramping from the tight bands (which can be alleviated by the application of a local anesthetic to the tube before or after banding).

The ring applicator consists of two concentric cylinders. Within the inner cylinder is a forceps for grasping, elevating, and retracting a segment of the tube. The silastic ring is stretched around the exposed end of the inner cylinder by means of a special ring loader and ring guide. The outer cylinder moves the ring from the inner cylinder on to the tube, a loop of which is held within the inner cylinder by the forceps.

The Silastic (Falope-Yoon) Ring

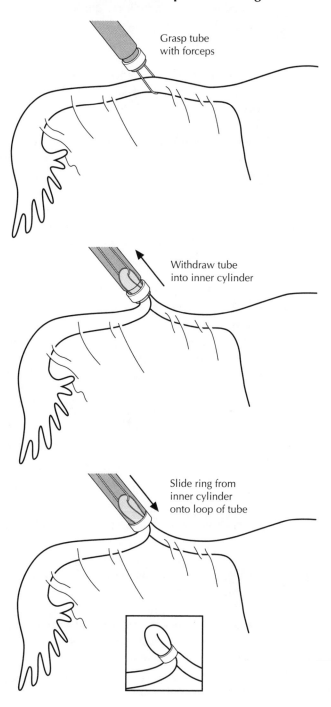

Grasp tube
with forceps

Withdraw tube
into inner cylinder

Slide ring from
inner cylinder
onto loop of tube

As with application of clips, the ring should be placed at the junction of the proximal and middle third of each fallopian tube. Once the tube is grasped, it is gently withdrawn into the inner cylinder by slowly squeezing the pistol-like handle of the applicator. A final strong pull is needed to slide the ring from the inner applicator cylinder onto the loop of tube. Necrosis occurs promptly and a 2–3 cm segment of the tube is destroyed. Failure rates are about 4 per 1,000 women at one year. [11]

Mesosalpingeal bleeding is the most common complication of silastic ring application. It usually occurs when the forceps grabs not only the tube but also a vascular fold of mesosalpinx. The mesosalpinx can also be torn on the edge of the stainless steel cylinder as the tube is drawn into the applicator. If bleeding is noted, application of the silastic band often controls it. If the placement of additional bands or electrocoagulation fails to stop bleeding, laparotomy may be required.

Silastic rings are occasionally placed on structures other than the tube. If this mistake is recognized, the band can usually be removed from the round ligament or mesosalpingeal folds by grasping the band with the tongs of the applicator and applying gradual, increasing traction. If a gentle attempt fails, removal is not necessary. If rings are inadvertently discharged into the peritoneal cavity, they can safely be left behind.

Patients should be prepared for the use of electrosurgical instruments in case bands or clips cannot be applied (because of adhesions or bleeding).

Minilaparotomy. Tubal ligation accomplished through a small suprapubic incision, "minilaparotomy," is the most frequent method of interval female sterilization around the world. In the U.S. and most of the developed world, laparoscopy is more popular, but minilaparotomy is gaining in favor because of its safety, simplicity, and adaptability to ambulatory surgical settings (particularly when local anesthesia is used).[20]

The fallopian tubes can be occluded through the minilaparotomy incision with bands or clips, but a simple Pomeroy-type tubal ligation is the method most commonly used. Patient characteristics such as obesity, previous pelvic infection, or previous surgery are the principal determinants of complications.[21]

Minilaparotomy is accomplished through an incision which usually measures 3–5 cm in length. Tubal ligation through a suprapubic incision can be accomplished for obese patients, but the incision will necessarily exceed the usual length. Forceful retraction increases the pain associated with the procedure and the time of recovery. For these reasons, we believe that minilaparotomy for ambulatory tubal occlusion should be limited to patients who are not obese (usually less than 150–160 pounds, 70 kg).

Patients who are likely to have adhesions from previous surgery or pelvic infection will probably have a shorter operating and recovery time (and less pain) with open laparoscopic tubal occlusion. In addition, the wide view provided by the laparoscope will make possible a precise description of the pelvic abnormalities which may be useful should the patient develop chronic pelvic pain or recurrent infection.

Tubal occlusion is difficult to accomplish through a minilaparotomy if the uterus is immobile. Laparoscopic tubal occlusion, on the other hand, does not require extreme uterine elevation or rotation, and is a better choice for a patient with a uterus fixed in position.

Counseling for Sterilization

All patients undergoing a surgical procedure for permanent contraception should be aware of the nature of the operation, its alternatives, efficacy, safety, and complications. The operation can be described using drawings or pelvic models, as well as films, slides, or video tapes. The description of the operation should emphasize its similarities to and differences from laparoscopy and pelvic surgery, especially hysterectomy or ovariectomy which may be confused with simple tubal ligation. Alternatives, including vasectomy, oral contraception, long-acting hormone methods, barrier methods, and IUDs should be specified. It should be emphasized to the patient that tubal ligation is not intended to be reversible, and that it cannot be guaranteed to prevent intrauterine or ectopic pregnancy. Informed consent is best obtained at a time when a patient is not distracted or distraught, for example, not immediately before or after a therapeutic abortion.

Sexuality. There is no detrimental effect on sexuality specifically due to sterilization procedures.[22] Indeed, sexual life is usually positively affected. Many couples are less inhibited and more spontaneous in love making when they don't have to worry about an unwanted pregnancy.

Menstrual Function. The effects on menstrual function are less clear, and therefore more difficult to explain. The first well-controlled studies of this issue demonstrated no change in menstrual patterns, volume, or pain.[23,24] Subsequently these same authors reported an increase in dysmenorrhea and changes in menstrual bleeding.[25,26] However, these authors failed to agree in their findings (a change found by one group was not confirmed by the other). Adding to the confusion, the incidence of hysterectomy for bleeding disorders was reported to be increased by some[27], but not by others.[28] These discordant reports do not make patient counseling about the long-term effects of tubal sterilization an easy task.

Extensive electrocoagulation of the fallopian tubes can change ovarian steroid production. Perhaps this is why menstrual changes were detected with longer (4 years) follow-up.[26] More studies with careful attention to the type of tubal occlusion procedure will be necessary. The best answer for now is that some women experience menstrual changes, but most do not.

Reversibility. An important objective of counseling is to help couples make the right decision about an irreversible decision to become sterile. The active participation of both spouses is a critical factor.[29] Not all couples are pleased following sterilization; in one series, 2% of U.S. women expressed regret one year later, and 2.7% after two years.[30] At the two year mark, the main factors associated with regret were age less than 30 and sterilization at the convenient time of a cesarean section. In Europe where tubal sterilization is less common, the most important risk factor for regret was an unstable marriage.[31] A change in marital status is undoubtedly an important reason for a desire to reverse sterilization.[32]

Young women in unstable relationships need special attention in counseling, and both partners should participate in the counseling. Furthermore, for many couples tubal occlusion at the time of cesarean section or immediately after a difficult labor and delivery is not the best time for the procedure.

It is important to know that sterilized women have not been observed to develop psychological problems at a greater than expected rate.[33,34]

Microsurgery for tubal reanastomosis is associated with excellent results if only a small segment of the tube has been damaged. Pregnancy rates correlate with the length of remaining tube, a length of 4 cm or more is optimal. Thus, the pregnancy rates are lowest with electrocoagulation, and reach 70–80% with clips, rings, and surgical methods such as the Pomeroy. [35] About 2 per 1,000 sterilized women will eventually undergo tubal reanastomosis. [32]

Male Sterilization: Vasectomy

Vasectomy is safer, easier, and less expensive than female sterilization.[36] Hematomas and infection occur rarely and are easily treated with heat, scrotal support, and antibiotics. Most men will develop sperm antibodies following vasectomy, but no long-term sequelae have been observed, including no increased risk of cardiovascular disease.[9] Adverse psychological and sexual effects have not been reported. Since the other constituents of semen are made downstream from the testes, men do not notice a decreased volume or velocity of ejaculate. Vasectomy reversal is associated with pregnancy rates greater than 50%. The prospect for pregnancy diminishes with time elapsed from vasectomy, decreasing significantly after 10 years.

Abortion

By 1980, legal abortion became the most common surgical procedure performed in the U.S. Public health authorities have demonstrated that the legalization of abortion reduced maternal morbidity and mortality more than any single development since the advent of antibiotics to treat puerperal infections and blood banking to treat hemorrhage. The number of American women reported as dying from abortion declined from nearly 300 deaths in 1961, to only 6 in 1985 (1 death for every 200,000 legal abortions).[37] For comparison, in 1985, the death rate for childbirth in the U.S. was 10 per 100,000 births, and for ectopic pregnancy, 1 per 2,000 cases.[37]

The most important determinants of abortion mortality are duration of gestation and type of anesthesia: later abortions and general anesthesia are more hazardous.[38]

Complications of First Trimester Abortion [39]

Major Complications (hospitalization required):

Retained tissue	1:3,617
Sepsis	1:4,722
Uterine perforation	1:10,625
Hemorrhage	1:14,166
Inability to complete	1:28,333
Tubal pregnancy	1:42,500

Minor Complications (managed as outpatient):

Mild infection	1:216
Re-aspiration, same day	1:553
Re-aspiration, later	1:596
Cervical stenosis	1:6,071
Cervical tear	1:9,444
Underestimated gestational age	1:15,454
Convulsion	1:25,086

As with mortality, morbidity rates vary primarily with duration of pregnancy, but other factors are important as well, including type of operation, age of patient, type of anesthesia, operator's skill, and method of cervical dilatation.

The possibility that abortion can result in longer-term complications has been examined in over 150 studies.[40] First trimester abortion by vacuum aspiration is not associated with any adverse consequences on the following: subsequent fertility, subsequent pregnancies, or the risk of ectopic pregnancy.[41–44] It is not yet certain if second trimester abortions or multiple first trimester abortions can affect the outcome of later pregnancies.

Pre-operative Care of Abortion Patients

The care of the patient who has decided to terminate a pregnancy begins with the diagnosis of intrauterine pregnancy and an accurate estimate of gestational age. Failure to accomplish this is the most common source of abortion complications and subsequent litigation. Tests for pregnancy, including vaginal ultrasound, should be employed when accuracy is difficult.

More than 85% of the abortions performed in the U.S. occur in the first trimester of pregnancy. Morbidity and mortality rates with first trimester abortions are approximately one-tenth those of later abortions. Nearly all women who want to terminate a pregnancy in the first trimester are good candidates for an outpatient procedure under local anesthesia. Possible exceptions include patients with severe cardiorespiratory disease, severe anemias or coagulopathies, mental disorders severe enough to preclude cooperation, and excessive concern about operative pain that is not alleviated by reassurance.

Abortions should not be undertaken for women who have known uterine anomalies or leiomyomata, or who have previously had difficult first trimester abortion procedures, unless ultrasonography is immediately available and the surgeon is experienced in its intraoperative use. Previous cesarean section or other pelvic surgery is not a contraindication to outpatient first trimester abortion.

Second trimester pregnancies can also be safely terminated in an outpatient setting, when the cervix has been dilated pre-operatively with osmotic tents and the uterus is evacuated by an experienced surgeon, preferably under sonographic guidance.[45,46]

Counseling Abortion Patients

Counseling has played a critical role in the development of efficient and acceptable abortion services.[47] Whether abortion is accomplished in a clinic, physician's office, or a surgical center, the functions of a counselor must be fulfilled to ensure quality patient care. These include help with decision making, provision of information about the procedure, obtaining informed consent, provision of emotional support for the patient and her family before, during, and after the operation, and providing information about contraception.[48] Referral opportunities should be provided for prenatal care or adoption for women who choose to carry an unplanned pregnancy to term. These responsibilities can be carried out by a physician, nurse, psychologist, social worker, or a trained lay person. An informed consent document should unequivocally state the possibilities of common adverse outcomes such as incomplete abortion, infection, uterine perforation, the need for laparotomy, ectopic pregnancy, and failed abortion. The counselor should document that all pre-operative responsibilities have been discharged.

Methods for First Trimester Abortions

The most widely used technique for first trimester abortions is vacuum curettage. The procedure is performed using local anesthesia (a paracervical block). Cervical dilatation is accomplished using tapered dilators (the Pratt dilators). Some surgeons recommend the preoperative insertion of cervical tents. These are osmotic dilators of dried seaweed or synthetic hydrophilic substances left in place from a few hours (synthetic) to overnight (seaweed).[49] After the procedure, the patient is observed for 1–2 hours before returning home.

In September, 1988, France and China approved the marketing of RU486 as an abortifacient. RU486 is a synthetic relative of the progestational agents in birth control pills. It acts primarily, but not totally, as an anti-progestational agent. RU486 is administered together with a prostaglandin analogue. The combination allows a reduction in dosage of both agents. When administered early in pregnancy, this medical treatment carries with it a success and complication rate similar to that achieved with vacuum curretage.[50] It is likely that abortion is the result of multiple actions. Although RU486 does not induce labor, it does open and soften the cervix (this may be an action secondary to prostaglandins). Its major action is its blockade of progesterone receptors in the endometrium. This leads to a disruption of the embryo and the production of prostaglandins. The disruption of the embryo and perhaps a direct action on the trophoblast leads to a decrease in HCG and a withdrawal of support from the corpus luteum. The success rate is dependent upon the length of pregnancy—the more dependent the pregnancy is upon progesterone from the corpus luteum, the more likely the progesterone antagonist, RU486, will result in abortion.

Complications of Abortions

Postoperative complications of elective abortions are classified as either immediate or delayed. Uterine perforation and uterine atony are examples of immediate complications. Delayed complications can occur several hours to several weeks after the operation. These usually present according to the major complaint: bleeding, pain, and continuing symptoms of pregnancy.

Patients should be informed of the 3 signs of possible complications: increased bleeding, pain, and fever. A telephone number should be provided for advice or questions at any time during the day or night.

Since the majority of abortion complications occur during the first week following an abortion, the postoperative visit is best scheduled during that first week. This is a good time to examine the patient for pelvic tenderness as a sign of endometritis or salpingitis, to assess uterine involution and bleeding, and to answer questions regarding contraception, sexually transmitted diseases, and return to sexual activity.

Bleeding. By far the most common cause of unusually heavy post abortal bleeding is retained products of conception. Rates in large series vary from 0.2 to 0.6%.[39] Patients with retained products of conception occasionally present several weeks after an abortion, but most report excessive bleeding within one week. Severe pain or pelvic tenderness suggests that infection is also present. Treatment is prompt aspiration of the uterus with the largest cannula that will pass the cervix.

Infection. Infection is sometimes marked by uterine bleeding, although without retained products of conception, the volume of blood loss is usually modest. Fever and uterine tenderness are the most common signs of post abortal endometritis, occurring in about 0.5% of cases.[39] Some studies indicate that prophylactic antibiotics reduce the risk of post abortal infection. Most clinicians agree that women at high risk for pelvic infection (for example, previous episodes of salpingitis or post abortal endometritis) benefit from the use of prophylactic antibiotics prior to abortion, but some believe that all abortion patients should have prophylactic antibiotics.[51] Doxycycline, 100 mg an hour before the procedure and 200 mg one-half hour afterwards is the most convenient and comprehensive regimen.[52] Metronidazole, 400 mg an hour before and 4 and 8 hours afterward, has also been used.[53]

Patients who present with uterine tenderness, fever, and bleeding require uterine re-aspiration as well as antibiotic treatment. Patients who have fevers above 38°C (101°F) and signs of peritoneal inflammation, as well as uterine tenderness, require hospitalization and intravenous antibiotics active against anaerobes, gonorrhea, and chlamydia. Outpatient treatment with doxycycline, 100 mg bid for 14 days, should be reserved for patients whose signs and symptoms are confined to the uterus.

Dysfunctional Uterine Bleeding Following Abortion. Women may present with uterine bleeding but without signs or symptoms of retained products of conception or infection. When these two diagnoses have been ruled out by absence of fever, a closed cervix, and a nontender uterus, the bleeding itself can be treated hormonally. Curettage is rarely necessary unless bleeding is excessive.

Ectopic Pregnancy. Failure to diagnose ectopic pregnancy at the time of therapeutic abortion can cause a patient to return with complaints of persistent bleeding with or without pelvic pain. Careful examination of the uterine aspirate for villi at the time of abortion should make a missed ectopic pregnancy an unusual cause of delayed bleeding. If, however, a patient presents with this possibility, quantitative measurement of chorionic gonadotropin and vaginal ultrasonography should be utilized for accurate diagnosis and management.

Cervical Stenosis. Patients who experience amenorrhea or hypomenorrhea and cyclic uterine pain after first trimester abortion may have stenosis of the internal os. This condition occurs in about 0.02% of cases, and is more common among women whose abortions are performed in the early first trimester with a minimum of cervical dilatation and a small diameter, flexible plastic cannula.[54] Possibly the tip of this type of cannula abrades the internal os and the minimal dilatation allows the abraded areas to heal in contact. The condition is easily treated with cervical dilatation with Pratt dilators under paracervical block.

Other Late Complications. Amenorrhea, usually without pain, can also be caused by Asherman's syndrome, destruction and scarification of the endometrium. This condition is very rare, and usually follows endometrial infection. This problem is best diagnosed and treated at hysteroscopy.

Sensitization of Rh negative women should be prevented. Approximately 4% of these women become sensitized following an induced abortion (the later the abortion the higher the proportion). Subsequent hemolytic disease of the newborn can be prevented by administering 50 micrograms of Rh immune globulin to all Rh negative, Du negative women undergoing early abortion. The standard dose is administered for second trimester abortion.

Abortion in the Second Trimester

Second trimester abortions can be accomplished surgically or medically. The surgical procedure is termed dilatation and evacuation (D & E). Several approaches have been utilized for the medical termination of pregnancy. These include the vaginal, intramuscular, or intraamniotic administration of prostaglandins and the intraamniotic injection of hypertonic saline or urea. The D & E procedure is safer and less expensive than the medical methods, and is better tolerated (and thus, preferred) by patients.[55,56]

The training, experience, and skills of the surgeon are the primary factors which limit the gestational age at which abortion can be safely performed. Most surgeons can assess these factors for themselves and establish a rational limit for gestational age. The attitudes of the staff, including counselors, administrators, and nurses, the availability of emergency support, such as a nearby hospital willing and able to accept the transfer of complicated cases, are also factors.

Advanced gestational age by itself incurs increased risks for all types of complications. These are multiplied when the duration of pregnancy is discovered, after beginning uterine evacuation, to be beyond the experience and skill of the surgeon or capacity of the equipment. Uterine perforation, infection, bleeding, amniotic fluid embolism, and anesthetic reactions are increased as gestational age increases.[45,55]

When errors in estimating gestational age require the surgeon to use unfamiliar instruments or techniques that are not frequently practiced, the increased duration of the procedure can cause problems.[57] Efforts to sedate or relieve pain by administering additional drugs increase the risk of toxic reactions or overdosage. If a change from local to general anesthesia is undertaken, the patient is at much greater risk of anesthetic complications. Finally, if complications caused by advanced gestational age necessitate transfer of the patient to physicians who are not familiar with uterine evacuation techniques, the patient may undergo unnecessarily extensive surgery, such as hysterectomy, with all the risks inherent in emergency procedures.

Pre-operative cervical dilatation with osmotic dilators makes first trimester abortion safer and easier, and is essential for second trimester abortion.[49] Local anesthesia instead of general anesthesia also makes abortion safer.[58,59] Some patients are not good candidates for surgical procedures of any kind under local anesthesia, and others may have special reasons to prefer that an abortion be performed under general anesthesia. Patient requests should be seriously considered, but the clinician also has a responsibility to inform the patient of the risks and benefits of local versus general anesthesia.

References

1. Mosher WD, Pratt WF, Contraceptive use in the United States, 1973–88, Advance data from vital and health statistics; No. 182, National Center for Health Statistics, Hyattsville, Maryland, 1990.

2. Mosher WD, Use of family planning services in the United States: 1982 and 1988, Advance data from vital and health statistics, No. 184, National Center for Health Statistics, Hyattsville, Maryland, 1990.

3. Henshaw SK, Van Vort J, Abortion services in the United States, 1987 and 1988, Fam Plann Persp 22:102, 1990.

4. Speert H, *Obstetric and Gynecologic Milestones*, The Macmillan Company, New York, 1958, pp 619–629.

5. Lungren SS, A case of cesarean section twice successfully performed on the same patient, with remarks on the time, indications, and details of the operation, Am J Obstet 14:78, 1881.

6. Centers for Disease Control, Surgical sterilization surveillance: Tubal sterilization 1976–1978, 1981.

7. Layde PM, Ory HW, Peterson HB, et al, The declining lengths of hospitalization for tubal sterilizations, JAMA 245:714, 1981.

8. Escobedo LG, Peterson HB, Grubb GS, Franks AL, Case fatality rates for tubal sterilization in U.S. hospitals, Am J Obstet Gynecol 160:147, 1989.

9. Peterson HB, Huber DH, Belker AM, Vasectomy: An appraisal for the obstetrician-gynecologist, Obstet Gynecol 76:568, 1990.

10. Trussell J, Hatcher RA, Cates W Jr, Stewart FH, Kost K, Contraceptive failure in the United States: An update, Stud Fam Plann 21:51, 1990.

11. Chi IC, Laufe L, Gardner SD, Tolbert M, An epidemiologic study of risk factors associated with pregnancy following female sterilizations, Am J Obstet Gynecol 136:768, 1980.

12. Cheng M, Wong YM, Rochat R, Ratnam SS, Sterilization failures in Singapore: An examination of ligation techniques and failure rates, Stud Fam Plann 8:109, 1977.

13. Lichter ED, Laff SP, Friedman EA, Value of routine dilation and curettage at the time of interval sterilization, Obstet Gynecol 67:763, 1986.

14. McCausland A, High rate of ectopic pregnancy following laparoscopic tubal coagulation failure, Am J Obstet Gynecol 136:977, 1980.

15. Chi IC, Laufe LE, Atwed R, Ectopic pregnancy following female sterilization procedures, Adv Plann Parenthood 16:52, 1981.

16. Miesfeld R, Gaarontans R, Moyers T, Vaginal tubal ligation. Is infection a significant risk? Am J Obstet Gynecol 137:183, 1980.

17. Population Information Program, Minilaparotomy and laparoscopy: Safe, effective, and widely used, Johns Hopkins University, Population Reports, C-9, 1985.

18. Centers for Disease Control, Deaths following female sterilization with unipolar electrocoagulating devices, MMWR 30:150, 1981.

19. Soderstrom RM, Levy BS, Engel T, Reducing bipolar sterilization failures, Obstet Gynecol 74:60, 1989.

20. McCann M, Cole L, Laparoscopy and minilaparotomy: Two major advances in female sterilization, Stud Fam Plann 11:119, 1980.

21. Layde PM, Peterson HB, Dicker RC, et al, Risk factors for complications of interval tubal sterilization by laparotomy, Obstet Gynecol 62:180, 1983.

22. Kjer J, Sexual adjustment to tubal sterilization, Eur J Obstet Gynecol 35:211, 1990.

23. Rulin MC, Turner JH, Dunworth R, Thompson D, Post tubal sterilization syndrome: A misnomer, Am J Obstet Gynecol 151:13, 1985.

24. DeStefano F, Huezo CM, Peterson HB, et al, Menstrual changes after tubal sterilization, Obstet Gynecol 62:673, 1983.

25. Rulin MC, Davidson AR, Philliber SG, Graves WL, Cushman LF, Changes in menstrual symptoms among sterilized and comparison women: A prospective study, Obstet Gynecol 79:749, 1989.

26. DeStefano F, Perlman J, Peterson HB, Diamond E, Long-term risk of menstrual disturbances after tubal sterilization, Am J Obstet Gynecol 152:835, 1985.

27. Kjer J, Knudsen L, Hysterectomy subsequent to laparoscopic sterilization, Eur J Obstet Gynecol 35:63, 1990.

28. Stergachis A, Shy KK, Gouthaus LC, Wagner EH, Hecht JA, Anderson G, Normand EH, Raboud J, Tubal sterilization and the long-term risk of hysterectomy, JAMA 264:2893, 1990.

29. Miller WB, Shain RN, Pasta DJ, Tubal sterilization or vasectomy: How do married couples make the decision? Fertil Steril 56:278, 1991.

30. Grubb G, Refoser H, Layde PM, Rubin GL, Regret after decision to have a tubal sterilization, Fertil Steril 44:248, 1985.

31. Vemer HM, Colla P, Schoot DC, Willensen WN, Bierkens PB, Rolland R, Women regretting their sterilization, Fertil Steril 46:724, 1986.

32. Wilcox LS, Chu SY, Peterson HB, Characteristics of women who considered or obtained tubal reanastomosis: Results from a prospective study of tubal sterilization, Obstet Gynecol 75:661, 1990.

33. Vessey M, Huggins G, Lawless M, et al, Tubal sterilization: Findings in a large prospective study, Br J Obstet Gynaecol 90:203, 1983.

34. W.H.O., Mental health and female sterilization: Report of a WHO collaborative study, J Biosc Sci 16:1, 1984.

35. Siegler AM, Hulka J, Peretz A, Reversibility of female sterilization, Fertil Steril 43:499, 1985.

36. Smith GL, Taylor GP, Smith KF, Comparative risks and costs of male and female sterilization, Am J Public Health 75:370, 1985.

37. Lawson H, Atrash HK, Safflas A, et al, Ectopic pregnancy surveillance, United States, 1970–1986, Abortion surveillances, 1984–1985. MMWR 38:11, 1989.

38. Buehler J, Schulz KF, Grimes DA, Hogue C, The risk of serious complications from induced abortion: Do personal characteristics make a difference? Am J Obstet Gynecol 153:14, 1985.

39. Hakim-Elahi E, Tovell HM, Burnhill MS, Complications of first trimester abortion: A report of 170,000 cases, Obstet Gynecol 76:929, 1990.

40. Hogue CJ, Impact of abortion on subsequent fecundity, Clin Obstet Gynecol 13:951, 1986.

41. Stubblefield P, Monson R, Schoenbaum S, et al, Fertility after induced abortion: A prospective follow-up study, Obstet Gynecol 62:186, 1984.

42. Daling J, Weiss N, Voigt L, et al, Tubal infertility in relation to prior induced abortion, Fertil Steril 43:389, 1985.

43. Schoenbaum S, Monson R, Stubblefield P, et al, Outcome of the delivery following an induced or spontaneous abortion, Am J Obstet Gynecol 136:19, 1980.

44. Daling J, Chow W, Weiss N, et al, Ectopic pregnancy in relation to previous induced abortion, JAMA 253:1005, 1985.

45. Peterson WF, Berry FN, Grace MR, Gulbranson CL, Second trimester abortion by dilatation and evacuation: An analysis of 11,747 cases, Obstet Gynecol 62:185, 1983.

46. Darney PD, Sweet RL, Routine intraoperative ultrasonography for second trimester abortion reduces incidence of uterine perforation, J Ultrasound Med 8:71, 1989.

47. Landy U, Lewit S, Administrative, counseling, and medical practices in National Abortion Federation facilities, Fam Plann Perspect 14:257, 1982.

48. Landy U, Abortion counselling—A new component of Medical care, Clin Obstet Gynecol 13:33, 1986.

49. Darney PD, Atkinson E, Hirabayashi K, Uterine perforation during second trimester abortion by cervical dilation and instrumental extraction: A review of 15 cases, Obstet Gynecol 75:441, 1990.

50. Silvestre L, Dubois C, Renault M, Rezvani Y, Baulieu EE, Ulmann A, Voluntary interruption of pregnancy with Mifepristone (RU 486) and a prostaglandin analogue, New Engl J Med 322:645, 1990.

51. Darj E, Stralin EB, Nilsson S, The prophylactic effect of doxycycline on postoperative infection rate after first trimester abortion, Obstet Gynecol 70:755, 1987.

52. Levallois P, Rioux JE, Prophylactic antibiotics for suction curettage abortion: Results of a clinical controlled trial, Am J Obstet Gynecol 158:100, 1988.

53. Heisterberg L, Petersen K, Metronidazole prophylaxis in elective first trimester abortion, Obstet Gynecol 65:371, 1985.

54. Hakim-Elahi E, Postabortal amenorrhea due to cervical stenosis, Obstet Gynecol 48:723, 1976.

55. Grimes DA, Schulz KF, Cates W Jr, Tyler CW, Midtrimester abortion by dilation and evacuation, New Engl J Med 296:1141, 1977.

56. Kafrissen M, Schulz K, Grimes D, Cates W Jr, Midtrimester abortion: Intra amniotic instillation of hyperosmolar urea and prostaglandin F2a v dilatation and evacuation, JAMA 251:916, 1984.

57. Darney PD, Dorward K, Cervical dilation before first-trimester abortion: A controlled comparison of meteneprost, laminaria and hypan, Obstet Gynecol 70:397, 1987.

58. Mackay T, Schulz K, Grimes D, Safety of local versus general anesthesia for second trimester dilatation and evacuation abortion, Obstet Gynecol 66:661, 1985.

59. Atrash HK, Check T, Hogue CJ, Legal abortion and general anesthesia, Am J Obstet Gynecol 158:420, 1988.

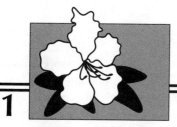

11

The Future of Contraception

INADEQUATE RESEARCH funding, political pressures, and product liability concerns represent a concert of forces which have slowed contraceptive development in the U.S.A. in the last decade. We predict, however, that in the coming years new contraceptive options will be forthcoming. The pressures of increasing population density are increasing, and attention is being directed to the development of new contraceptives.[1] New methods require the combined efforts of individuals, scientists, and policymakers. We believe our society will respond to our needs. We already can see emerging and promising new developments.

Biodegradable Implants

Biodegradable implants deliver sustained levels of progestin for variable periods of time from a vehicle that dissolves in body tissues. The utility of implant contraception would be improved by the elimination of the need for surgical removal. Two types are currently under evaluation: Capronor and norethindrone pellets.

Capronor

Capronor is a single capsule, biodegradable, levonorgestrel-releasing subdermal implant composed of the polymer E-caprolactone. Implants measure 0.24 cm in diameter and either 2.5 or 4 cm in length, providing contraception for one year. The shorter capsule contains 16 mg levonorgestrel, and the longer contains 26 mg.

297

Levonorgestrel escapes from caprolactone at a rate 10 times faster than from Silastic. The shorter implant maintains circulating levels of levonorgestrel of 0.2–0.3 ng/ml, while the longer implant maintains higher levels equivalent to those found in Norplant users. The longer capsule suppresses ovulation in a higher proportion (about 50%) of cycles than reported with Norplant, but the shorter implant allows ovulation in most users.[2] The higher release rate allows the use of a smaller implant. Experience is thus far too limited to report pregnancy rates, but the longer implant should provide contraception comparable to Norplant.

When exposed to tissue fluids, E-caprolactone slowly breaks down into E-hydroxycaproic acid, then finally to carbon dioxide and water. The capsule remains intact during the first 12 months of use, allowing easy removal. After 12 months, the capsule begins to disappear.

Capronor shares the advantages of Norplant with convenience of use and few metabolic effects. There is no adverse impact on the lipoprotein profile. Removal is easier and quicker. The disadvantages are also similar to Norplant: changes in menstrual patterns and the other side effects typical of low-dose, continuous progestin systems. Biodegradable implants could continue to release small, noncontraceptive amounts of hormone after their period of use as a contraceptive had expired. Although it is unlikely that such low serum levels of progestin would be harmful to users or to their pregnancies, this question needs to be resolved. The degrading implants can be removed in the event of pregnancy.

Insertion and Removal. Capronor insertions and removals are simple and rapid. After local anesthesia is injected at the insertion site in the skin of the upper inner arm, a single-use, thin-walled, stainless steel trocar is used to pierce the skin. An incision is not required. The trocar is advanced just under the skin, as with Norplant insertions, to a mark near the handle. The trocar is then retracted back into the handle so that the stationary obturator holds the implant in its position under the skin. An adhesive strip and pressure dressing are applied as with Norplant. The procedure takes about 1 minute.

When Capronor requires removal, the distal tip of the implant is identified with digital pressure. A wheal of local anesthetic is raised at the site and a 2–3 mm skin incision is made at the distal tip of the implant. The fibrous sheath covering the implant is opened and the implant is extruded using digital pressure until it can be grasped and pulled out. The procedure takes about 3 minutes. Instruments are not required for any Capronor removals. At completion, an adhesive strip is used to close the incision and a small bandage is applied over the wound.

Other Implants

The newer progestins (desogestrel, gestodene, and norgestimate) are even more potent than levonorgestrel and could prove useful in contraceptive implants. An example is "Implanon," a single ethinyl vinyl acetate capsule about 4 cm long, containing 3 keto desogestrel. Implanon is designed to provide contraception from 1–2 years after which the implant should be removed. Clinical trials are underway.

Nearer completion of clinical trials is a two implant "Norplant II" system using levonorgestrel suspended in a silastic matrix and covered with a silastic membrane. Like the 6 capsule Norplant and the single capsule Implanon, Norplant II should also be removed when serum levonorgestrel levels are too low for contraception, at least 3 years after insertion, but possibly as long as 5 years.

Norethindrone Pellets

Biodegradable subdermal norethindrone pellets are expected to maintain circulating concentrations of this progestin at contraceptive levels for 12–18 months, and to completely disappear within 24 months. The pellets are composed of 10% pure cholesterol and 90% norethindrone, and are about the size of a grain of rice. This method is currently under development to determine the correct size and number of pellets and the cholesterol/hormone ratio necessary to obtain the release rates which provide contraception.

Preliminary trials of 2, 3, and 4 pellets have demonstrated that bleeding patterns are disrupted during the first few months of use, then return to normal patterns. Users of 4 pellets are more likely to be amenorrheic and anovulatory. As with Norplant, the circulating levels of progestin are too low to produce metabolic effects.

Injectable Norethindrone Microspheres

Microspheres or microcapsules which provide contraception consist of a biodegradable copolymer and one or more hormones. Like other injectable contraceptive methods, such as Depo-Provera, they are easy to administer and are highly effective. Unlike implants, injectables do not require surgical skills of the clinician and can be discontinued by the patient simply by declining to have another injection. Unlike implants, the microspheres cannot be removed once they are injected; if a woman experiences side effects or becomes pregnant, she must continue use of the method until the hormone is completely metabolized. For this reason, the duration of action of the norethindrone capsules has been limited to a few months.

The carrier of the microsphere is composed of a polymer commonly used in biodegradable suture, poly-dl-lactide-co-glycolide. The size of the microspheres varies from 0.06 to 0.1 mm in diameter, and each is composed of about 50% norethindrone dispersed within the polymer.[3,4] The release of norethindrone occurs initially by diffusion and later by degradation of the carrier. The size of the microspheres, the amount of hormone contained within the carrier, and the quantity of microspheres delivered by injection determine the daily dose of norethindrone delivered. Injections currently under evaluation contain a total dose of either 65 mg or 100 mg norethindrone, and the amount released daily is approximately the same as that delivered by low-dose oral contraception, but circulating levels are, of course, more stable.

The microspheres come preloaded in a syringe and are put into suspension with the addition of 2.5 ml of dextran diluent and vigorously agitated. The mixture must be shaken until all of the microspheres are in suspension, and again immediately prior to injection. The microspheres are deposited in the gluteal muscle using a 21-gauge needle and Z-track intramuscular injection technique.

As with other progestin-only methods of contraception, menstrual changes occur and are the most common cause of discontinuation during the first year of use. Users may experience amenorrhea or persistent or irregular spotting or bleeding.

In contrast to Depo-Provera, hormone levels decline rapidly after the microspheres have degraded, so that contraceptive effectiveness ends promptly at the predicted time. Most users will resume ovulatory cycles within 2–3 months after the predicted duration of the injection. If pregnancy occurs shortly after expiration of the norethindrone microspheres, the fetus will not be exposed to significant levels of norethindrone.

Microsphere preparations containing norethindrone combined with ethinyl estradiol are also under development. It is hoped that the addition of estrogen at a low dose will lead to fewer menstrual irregularities.

Intravaginal Rings

The search for a highly effective contraceptive system which would rely on the user for initiation and termination led to the development of steroid-releasing vaginal rings. The contraceptive action of vaginal rings is provided by the sustained release of hormones (either progestin alone or in combination with estrogen) which are absorbed through the lining of the vaginal vault. Progestin-only rings induce the usual changes in endometrium and cervical mucus associated with exposure to low, constant levels of progestin. Rings containing estrogen and a progestin also inhibit ovulation.

The biggest advantage of the vaginal ring over other long-acting, sustained-release methods is the ease with which the patient herself can both place the ring and remove it from the vagina. The vaginal ring is not a coitus-related method of contraception, a major disadvantage of other vaginal methods. The levonorgestrel-containing ring can be removed from the vagina for up to 24 hours without decreased effectiveness. In clinical trials, women reported removing rings prior to intercourse because their partners could feel them.

The rings have several disadvantages. the vaginal ring has a lower efficacy rate than injectables, implants, or medicated IUDs. As with other progestin-only methods, use of vaginal rings causes irregular bleeding patterns. Additional reasons for discontinuation include vaginal discharge, irritation, and infection of the vaginal vault, expulsion with urination or defecation (in 15–20% of users), discomfort with intercourse, and difficult insertion or removal.

301

Levonorgestrel Rings

The levonorgestrel vaginal ring was developed by the World Health Organization and has been undergoing evaluation since 1972. The device consists of an inner core containing 6 mg levonorgestrel combined with Silastic, and an outer Silastic shell measuring 55.6 mm in diameter with a cross-sectional diameter of 9.5 mm. This ring releases about 20 µg levonorgestrel per day, and can be left in place providing continuous contraception for 3 months. It prevents ovulation in 20–50% of cycles. A pregnancy rate of 3.5 per 100 woman-years has been reported.[5] The most frequent cause for discontinuation is menstrual irregularity. Expulsion increases with increasing age, body weight, and parity.

A new type of progestin-only vaginal ring containing 3-keto-desogestrel is currently under development.[6]

Progesterone Rings

The natural progesterone ring was developed by the Population Council for use during lactation. This ring releases 5–10 mg progesterone daily, and can provide continuous protection for 3 months.

Progestin and Estrogen Rings

A vaginal ring containing 50 mg ethinyl estradiol and 100 mg levonorgestrel releases 250–290 µg of the estrogen and 150–180 µg of the progestin per cycle. The ring is placed in the vagina on day 7 of the cycle and it is removed 21 days later to allow menstruation. Pregnancy rates ranged from 0.7 to 1.8 per 100 woman-years.[7]

Vaginal rings have been studied delivering norethindrone acetate and different doses of ethinyl estradiol. These rings are left in the vagina only 12 hours daily, and if enough estrogen is given, ovulation can be inhibited.

The addition of estrogen was expected to reduce the frequency of bleeding problems. However, despite the addition of estrogen, some women still experience breakthrough bleeding. Expulsion of the ring continues to be a common problem, as well as interference with coitus.

Intracervical Devices

Intracervical devices are promising sustained release vehicles for contraceptive progestins. Unnoticed expulsions have increased the failure rate and experimental modification continues.[8]

302

There is a levonorgestrel-releasing intracervical device which is still under development. Thus far, there has been a relatively high expulsion rate in the first year of use, and therefore, a high pregnancy rate.

GnRH Agonists and Antagonists

Both GnRH agonists and antagonists can provide ovarian suppression. There are two major problems which must be resolved. Partial suppression can lead to unopposed endogenous estrogen exposure with subsequent bleeding and endometrial complications. Total suppression yields a clinically significant hypoestrogenic state with all of the consequences of estrogen deprivation. In addition, since they cannot be administered orally, periodic administration with vehicles such as biodegradable microcapsules or silastic implants must be considered.

This approach has been studied in men as well. Invididual variability in response is a problem. In addition, testosterone must be administered intramuscularly in order to maintain libido.

This class of contraceptive agents is many years away from general use.

Immunologic Methods

The development of a vaccine against human chorionic gonadotropin (HCG) has been pursued for many years.[9] The obstacle has been the achievement of reliable levels of circulating antibodies, and work continues in an effort to develop appropriate adjuvants. Vaccines against other hormones, sperm antigens, and ovum antigens are in early stages of development, many years from clinical trials.

Male Contraception

A reversible method of contraception for men has been sought for years. Hormonal contraception for men is inherently a difficult physiologic problem because, unlike cyclic ovulation in women, spermatogenesis is continuous.[10] Investigational approaches to inhibit production of sperm include the administration of sex steroids, the use of GnRH analogs, and the administration of gossypol, a derivative of cotton seed oil.

303

The sex steroids reduce testosterone synthesis which leads to loss of libido and development of female secondary sexual characteristics. Furthermore, despite the use of large doses, sperm counts are not adequately reduced in all subjects. GnRH analogs also decrease the endogenous synthesis of testosterone, and supplemental testosterone must be provided.

Gossypol effectively decreases sperm counts to contraceptive levels, apparently by incapacitating the sperm producing cells. Gossypol pills are taken daily for 2 months until sperm are no longer observed in the ejaculate, and then the pills are taken weekly. Fertility returns to normal 3 months after discontinuation. Although the experience in China has been largely positive, animal studies in the U.S. indicate that gossypol, or contaminants of the preparation, are toxic. Analogs of gossypol may offer potential but are years away from development.

References

1. Mastroianni L Jr, Donaldson PJ, Kane TT, editors, *Developing New Contraceptives: Obstacles and Opportunities,* National Academy Press, Washington, DC, 1990.

2. Darney P, Monroe S, Klaisel C, Alvardo A, Clinical evaluation of the Capronor contraceptive implant: Preliminary report, Am J Obstet Gynecol 160:1292, 1989.

3. Singh M, Saxena BB, Graver R, Ledger WJ, Contraceptive efficacy of norethindrone encapuslated in injectable biodegradable poly-dl-lactide-co-glycolide microspheres: Phase II clinical study, Fertil Steril 52:973, 1989.

4. Beck L, Pope V, Long-acting injectable norethisterone contraceptive system: Review of clinical studies, Res Front Fertil Reg 3:1, 1984

5. WHO Task Force on Long-Acting Systemic Agents for Fertility Regulation, Microdose intravaginal levonorgestrel contraception: A multicentre clinical trial, Contraception 41:105,125,143,151, 1990.

6. Jackson R, Newton R, Pharmacodynamics of a contraceptive vaginal ring releasing 3-keto-desogestrel, Contraception 39:653, 1989.

7. Sivin I, Mishell D, Victor A, Diaz S, Alvarez-Sanchez F, Nielsen MC, et al, A multicenter study of levonorgestrel-estradiol contraceptive vaginal rings: 1. Use effectiveness: An international comparative trial, Contraception 24:341, 1981.

8. Ratsula K, Toivonen J, Lahteenmaki P, Luukkainen T, Plasma levonorgestrel levels and ovarian function during the use of a levonorgestrel-releasing intracervical contraceptive device, Contraception 39:195, 1989.

9. Jones WR, Bradley J, Judd SJ, Denholm EH, Ing RM, Mueller VW, Powell J, Griffin PD, Stevens VS, Phase I clinical trial of a World Health Organization birth control vaccine, Lancet i:1295, 1988.

10. Winters SJ, Marshall GR, Hormonally-based male contraceptives: Will they ever be a reality? J Clin Endocrinol Metab 73:464A, 1991.

12

Commonly Encountered Problems

A VISIT TO a clinician for the initiation or monitoring of
contraception provides an opportunity for preventive health
care. Asymptomatic problems, especially STDs, can and
should be detected. Furthermore, a relationship can be established
which will lead the patient to turn to the clinician when a problem
develops. In this chapter, we offer a brief, but accurate and effective,
guide to the management of commonly encountered clinical problems.

Vulvovaginitis

The Ecosystem

The vaginal environment is a dynamic system influenced by the
secretions of the epithelial cells, the pH, the hormonal milieu,
trauma, coitus, and the microbial flora.[1] In an estrogen-supported
vagina, the superficial epithelial cells have a high glycogen content.
The normal flora of the vagina utilize this rich supply of glycogen, and
as a result of the organic acids produced, the normal pH of the vagina
is acidic (pH 3.8–4.2). This acidic pH inhibits the overgrowth of
pathogens. The cervical mucus and the menstrual flow are alkaline,
providing better growth media for pathogens. Coitus and sexual
excitement also raise the vaginal pH and can predispose to vaginitis.

Candidiasis

Candida organisms grow well in the normal acidic pH of the vagina. Control of their growth depends heavily upon the presence of the other organisms in the normal vaginal flora. The disruption of the normal pH or the normal flora (e.g with the use of broad-spectrum antibiotics or immunosuppressive agents) allows the growth of foreign bacteria or the overgrowth of *Candida. Candida* species are opportunists; their growth to the point of vaginitis follows escape from inhibition by the normal flora. *Candida albicans* is the most common fungus, with *Candida glabrata* a distant second. *C. glabrata,* as with other *Candida* species, is more resistant to the usual treatment, but more sensitive to gentian violet. *Candida* species other than albicans are probably associated with chronicity and recurrence.

Symptoms. The major complaint is almost always pruritus, followed by burning and dysuria, and a vaginal discharge. Burning after intercourse is a characteristic symptom.

Discharge. The discharge, classically thick, white or yellow and curdlike, is not always prominent. It usually has a noticeable odor.

Diagnosis. An erythematous (sometimes shiny) appearance of the vagina and vulva is the usual finding. When found on the vulva, *Candida* are always present in the vagina and require intravaginal treatment. The vaginal pH is 4.0 to 4.5. *Note: If the pH is 4.5 or less, the patient either has Candida or a normal discharge. If symptoms are present, an infection with Candida is inevitably present.* The standard diagnostic tool consists of the vaginal smear, both the saline smear (to detect other pathogens) and the KOH smear (to lyse cellular material and allow *Candida* to stand out). The microscopic examination reveals budding filaments and spores with *C. albicans,* while only spores will be seen with *C. glabrata.*

The smears are often unrewarding, and in obvious contrast to the presenting complaints. Empiric treatment is worthwhile, but it is helpful to have tubes of Nickerson's media in the office. Inoculation and culture at room temperature will yield a definitive answer within a day or two. However, a sufficient number of organisms can be present to yield a recurrent infection but at the same time be insufficient to produce a colony on culture. Furthermore, significant infection can be present with minimal discharge and a normal-appearing vagina.

Treatment. The first line of treatment consists of one of the imidazole drugs or terconazole, used as vaginal creams or suppositories. While 3-day courses of treatment (2 suppositories qhs) have become popular and their effectiveness supported by clinical trials, clinical experience still indicates that longer treatment schedules (administration bid for 7–14 days) are more effective with lower recurrence rates.

As a last resort, an old tried and true treatment is recommended for resistant and recurrent *Candida* infections: gentian violet applied topically. The cervix, vagina, introitus, and inner vulva are painted with a 1% aqueous solution of gentian violet; residual liquid should be removed. Gentian violet impregnated in tampons or as a vaginal suppository is not as effective. Repeat treatment need not be more frequent than weekly, and usually no more than once or twice. It is equally effective against *C. albicans* and *C. glabrata.* The messy nature of this treatment is well accepted by patients in return for its rapid and effective results. The main problem is a stubborn stain on clothing, so be careful (ammonia and alcohol are only partially effective in removing stains, but the stains disappear with washing in bleach).

What to do for really resistant and recurrent cases? First make sure that other contributing factors are recognized and if possible eliminated or controlled. This includes diabetes mellitus, the use of antibiotics, oral-genital contact, and immune suppression. Then use continuous therapy, for 3–4 weeks. In addition, the male partner should be given an imidazole cream to use daily during the woman's period of treatment. It is not absolutely certain that treatment of a partner is helpful, but there is a high colonization rate with the same species in consorts of women with recurrent infections. For that reason, in extreme cases, both partners should be treated with an oral agent (fluconazole 100 mg daily for 3 days) to decrease the candidal reservoir in the gastrointestinal tract and the oral cavity as well as for its systemic action.[2] For the really recalcitrant chronic problem, provide the patient with long-term antifungal suppression, give ketoconazole, half a tablet (100 mg) daily for 6–12 months.[3] But note, liver enzymes must be monitored with long-term ketoconazole therapy. Fluconazole may be less likely to cause liver effects, and therefore 50 mg given daily for 6–12 months may be preferable to ketoconazole. Because this is not certain, to be on the safe side, liver enzymes should also be monitored with fluconazole long-term treatment. Finally, cryo treatment of the cervix should be given empirical consideration. Routine laundering does not destroy yeast.

In recalcitrant cases, it is worth treating underwear, either by boiling, soaking overnight in bleach, or exposure in a high-intensity microwave oven for 5 minutes.

Bacterial Vaginosis

In 1984, a new term was introduced, bacterial vaginosis. This condition is a bacterial vaginitis due to a variety of bacteria, including *Gardnerella vaginalis* (previously called *Hemophilus vaginalis* and *Corynebacterium vaginale*), as well as a newly recognized anaerobic rod named *Mobiluncus*. The prevalence of *G. vaginalis* in symptomatic and asymptomatic women has cast doubt on its etiologic significance as a single agent of infection. Bacterial vaginosis probably represents mixed infections due to an overgrowth of naturally occurring flora, including *G. vaginalis* and *Mobiluncus*, as well as anaerobes of the *Bacteroides* and *Peptococcus* species.

Symptoms. This infection is associated with a characteristic fishy odor due to the presence of amines produced by anaerobic bacteria in an alkaline vagina. Thus this odor may be noticed following intercourse with the introduction of alkaline semen.

Discharge. The discharge is thin, gray and homogeneous (and sometimes frothy).

Diagnosis. The vagina shows little inflammatory response because there is no invasion of the vaginal tissue (thus the term vaginosis rather than vaginitis), and hence, there are no complaints of pruritus or burning. The pH is 4.5 to 6.0. "Clue cells" are vaginal epithelial cells which appear intensely stippled with coccobacilli as the numerous bacteria that are present attach themselves to the surfaces of sloughed epithelial cells. They are no longer considered to be pathognomonic for *G. vaginalis,* however clue cells are an indicator of pathogenic bacterial vaginosis.

Treatment. The most effective treatment is metronidazole (500 mg bid for 7 days). Intolerance to alcohol while on metronidazole is a well-recognized side effect. The single dose method is definitely less effective. Clindamycin, 300 mg tid for 7 days, is also effective. Oral ampicillin or Keflex can be utilized (500 mg qid for 7 days), but effectiveness is reduced (50–65%). In patients with frequent recurrence, try using the 2% clindamycin cream (available as a preparation for acne) given intravaginally for 7 nights. An old standard, sulfa vaginal creams, is now known to be totally ineffective.[4] Metronidazole treatment of the partner is probably worthwhile with multiple recurrent infections, although studies on the effectiveness of this treatment have not reached consistent conclusions.

Trichomonas Vaginitis

Trichomonas vaginalis lives quietly in the paraurethral glands, seeding the vagina, and growing optimally in an alkaline pH.[5]

Symptoms. The cardinal symptom is a discharge, and sometimes urinary symptoms are caused by trichomonads. Itching and burning are more characteristic of *Candida*, but can occur with *Trichomonas* infection.

Discharge. The discharge is usually copious, malodorous, white, gray, or greenish. It is usually, but not always, frothy due to the carbon dioxide produced by the organisms.

Diagnosis. The vagina is erythematous. The pH is between 5 and 7. With a pH exceeding 6.0, an infection is almost always due to trichomonads. Those conditions associated with bacterial infections also encourage the growth of trichomonads. The traditional wet mount examination is insensitive, positive only 60% of the time in women with culture-proven infections. New office methods utilizing monoclonal antibodies are superior for accuracy of diagnosis.[6] Until such methods are widely available, there is room for empirical treatment. Indeed, a course of empirical treatment will be more cost effective than repeated efforts at trying to establish a specific diagnosis. It is further worth noting that the identification of trichomonads on Pap smear is not always acccurate, and an active infection may not be present.

Treatment. The treatment of choice is metronidazole given either in a short course to both partners (4 tablets, 1000 mg, in the AM, repeated once in the PM) or in a longer course (500 mg bid for 7 days). For recurrent cases resistant to treatment, consider high dose treatment (500 mg qid or 1000 mg bid, plus 500 mg bid given vaginally). The main toxicity risk is peripheral neuropathy. Minor side effects consist of a metallic taste and occasionally vomiting or diarrhea, all of which can by aggravated by alcohol ingestion. For those patients who cannot take metronidazole, topical treatment for 14 days should be prescribed, utilizing Vagisec suppositories or douche.

Pap Smear Comparison Chart

Old System	CIN System	Bethesda Reporting System				Recommend
I	Negative	Within normal limits				Routine follow-up
II	Negative	Reactive and reparative changes				Repeat smear or colposcopic examination
		Atypical squamous cells of undetermined significance				
		Atypical glandular cells of undetermined significance				
III	CIN-1	Squamous intraepithelial lesions (SIL)	Low grade	Changes associated with HPV (Condyloma)		Colposcopic examination and biopsy
				Mild dysplasia		Consider repeat smear if the smear is less than optimal
	CIN-2		High grade	Moderate dysplasia		
IV	CIN-3			Severe dysplasia or CIS		
V	Invasive	Malignant				Appropriate biopsy

Abnormal Pap Smears

The response to an abnormal Pap smear is relatively straightforward: an abnormal Pap smear requires colposcopic examination and appropriate biopsy. One word of caution—if the cytology laboratory does not report the presence of endocervical cells, the Pap smear must be repeated, being sure to use an endocervical brush. The failure to report endocervical cells is an important medical-legal issue if a Pap smear proves to be falsely negative.

Urinary Tract Infections

Clinical studies have generally supported empiric treatment for acute, uncomplicated urinary tract infections. From a cost effective point of view, it is acceptable to omit a culture in this circumstance. The drugs of choice are trimethoprim, trimethoprim/sulfamethoxazole, nitrofurantoin, or sulfa. Ampicillin is not recommended for first-line therapy.

It is important to identify patients with recurrent infections because of the significant risk of renal impairment. Women with recurrent infections should have urologic evaluation, including urography and cystoscopy, to identify correctable causes for reinfection, e.g. an urethral diverticulum. The urethral diverticulum is probably an acquired problem following trauma, catheterization, labor and delivery, or infections. The classic symptoms are dysuria, post voiding dribbling, and a purulent exudate expressible from the urethra. Surgical repair is necessary.

A midstream clean catch specimen which yields a positive result is sufficient for accurate diagnosis and management. The traditional requirement for a colony count of 100,000 or more per ml is no longer acceptable. Lower counts (as low as 100/ml) can be associated with significant infections.

Recurrent reinfection should be given a course of low-dose prophylaxis (maintained for at least 6 months).[7] An agent must be used that has no risk of causing resistance in the fecal flora.

Agents for Low-Dose Prophylaxis
1. Nitrofurantoin 100 mg qhs.
2. Cephalexin 250 mg qhs.
3. Trimethoprim-sulfamethoxazole (Bactrim, Cotrim, Septra) 40–200 mg qhs or trimethoprim 50 mg qhs.
4. Cinoxacin 250–500 mg qhs.

For difficult, recalcitrant cases, the patient can be educated to utilize self-start therapy. Treatment follows the demonstration of infection with one of the home testing kits. A 3 day full dose, empirical broad spectrum antimicrobial agent is used. Full doses of nitrofurantoin, cinoxacin, or norfloxacin are recommended. Ampicillin, tetracycline, sulfisoxazole, and cephalexin all should be avoided because of the propensity for resistant bacteria. Bacteriuria persistent 10 days after treatment requires follow-up evaluation.

Some patients have recurrent urinary tract infections that are related to sexual intercourse. It is worth trying the prophylactic administration of a single dose of an antibiotic postcoitally.

Mastalgia

The cyclic occurrence of breast discomfort is usually associated with dysplastic, benign histologic changes in the breast. Medical treatment of mastalgia has historically included a bewildering array of options. Several are of questionable value. Diuretics have little impact, and thyroid hormone replacement is indicated only when hypothyroidism is documented. Steroid hormone treatment has been tried in many combinations, mostly unsupported by controlled studies. An old favorite, with many years of clinical experience testifying to its effectiveness, is testosterone. One must be careful, however, to avoid virilizing doses. A good practice is to start with small doses, such as 5 mg methyltestosterone every other day during the time of discomfort. In recent years, however, these methods have been supplanted by several new approaches.

Danazol in a dose of 200 mg/day is effective in relieving discomfort as well as decreasing nodularity of the breast.[8] A daily dose is recommended for a period of 6 months. This treatment may achieve long-term resolution of the histologic changes in addition to the clinical improvement, however there is no evidence that treatment ameliorates atypical epithelial changes and reduces the risk of cancer. Doses below 400 mg daily do not assure inhibition of ovulation, and a method of effective contraception is necessary because of possible teratologic effects of the drug. Significant improvement has been noted with vitamin E, 600 units/day of the synthetic tocopheral acetate. No side effects have been noted, and the mechanism of action is unknown. Bromocriptine (2.5–5.0 mg/day) and antiestrogens such as tamoxifen (20 mg daily) are also effective for treating mammary discomfort and benign disease.[8,9]

Clinical observations had suggested that abstinence from methylxanthines leads to resolution of symptoms. Methylxanthines are present in coffee, tea, chocolate, and cola drinks. In controlled studies, however, a significant placebo response rate (30–40%) has been observed. Careful assessments of this relationship have failed to demonstrate a link between methylxanthine use and mastalgia, mammographic changes, or atypia (premalignant tissue changes).[10-12]

Galactorrhea

Galactorrhea refers to the mammary secretion of a milky fluid which is nonphysiologic in that it is inappropriate (not immediately related to pregnancy or the needs of a child), persistent, and sometimes excessive. Although usually white or clear, the color may be yellow or even green. In the latter circumstance, local breast disease also should be considered. To elicit breast secretion, pressure should be applied to all sections of the breast beginning at the base of the breast and working up toward the nipple. The quantity of secretion is not an important criterion. Any galactorrhea demands evaluation in a nulliparous woman, and, if at least 12 months have elapsed since the last pregnancy or weaning in a parous woman. Galactorrhea can involve both breasts, or just one breast. Amenorrhea does not necessarily accompany galactorrhea, even in the most serious provocative disorders.

Diagnosis

The differential diagnosis of galactorrhea syndromes is a difficult and complex clinical challenge. The difficulty arises from the multiple factors involved in the control of prolactin release. Before proceeding, it would be useful to reemphasize the mechanisms controlling prolactin secretion. In most pathophysiologic systems the final common pathway leading to galactorrhea is an inappropriate augmentation of prolactin release. Prolactin is under a chronic tonic inhibition due to the hypothalamic secretion into the pituitary portal system of a prolactin inhibiting factor (PIF). It is strongly believed that PIF is the neurotransmitter, dopamine. The following considerations are important:

1. Excessive estrogen (e.g. combined oral contraceptives) can lead to milk secretion via hypothalamic suppression, causing reduction of PIF and release of pituitary prolactin. Galactorrhea developing during oral contraceptive administration is most noticeable during the days free of medication (when the steroids are cleared from the body and the prolactin interfering action of the estrogen and progestin on the breast wanes). Galactorrhea caused by excessive estrogen disappears within 3–6 months after discontinuing medication.

This is now a rare occurrence with the lower dose pills. A longitudinal study of 126 women did demonstrate a 22% increase in prolactin values over mean control levels, but the response to low dose oral contraceptives was not out of the normal range.[13]

2. Prolonged intensive suckling can also release prolactin, via hypothalamic reduction of PIF. Similarly, thoracotomy scars, cervical spinal lesions, and herpes zoster can induce prolactin release by activating the afferent sensory neural arc, thereby simulating suckling.

3. A variety of drugs can also inhibit hypothalamic PIF. There are nearly 100 phenothiazine derivatives with indirect mammotropic activity of this type. In addition, there are many phenothiazine-like compounds, reserpine derivatives, amphetamines, and an unknown variety of other drugs (opiates, diazepams, butyrophenones, a-methyldopa, and tricyclic antidepressants) which can initiate galactorrhea via hypothalamic suppression. The final action of these compounds is either to deplete dopamine levels or to block dopamine receptors. Prolactin is uniformly elevated (but usually less than 100 ng/ml) in patients on therapeutic amounts of phenothiazines. Approximately 30–50% will exhibit galactorrhea which should not persist beyond 3–6 months after drug treatment is discontinued.

4. Stresses can inhibit hypothalamic PIF, thereby inducing prolactin secretion and galactorrhea. Trauma, surgical procedures, and anesthesia can be seen in temporal relation to the onset of galactorrhea.

5. Hypothalamic lesions, stalk lesions, or stalk compression (events that physically reduce production or delivery of PIF to the pituitary) allow release of excess prolactin leading to galactorrhea.

6. Hypothyroidism can be associated with galactorrhea. With diminished circulating levels of thyroid hormone, hypothalamic thyroid releasing hormone (TRH) is produced in excess and acts as a prolactin releasing hormone (PRH) to release prolactin from the pituitary. Reversal with thyroid hormone is strong circumstantial evidence to support the conclusion that TRH stimulates prolactin secretion. Prolactin levels associated

with primary hypothyroidism are less than 100 ng/ml.

7. Increased prolactin release may be a consequence of prolactin elaboration and secretion from pituitary tumors which function independently of the otherwise appropriate restraints exerted by PIF from a normally functioning hypothalamus. This potentially dangerous tumor, which has endocrine, neurologic, and ophthalmologic liabilities that can be disabling, makes the differential diagnosis of persistent galactorrhea a major clinical challenge. Beyond producing prolactin, the tumor may also suppress pituitary parenchyma by expansion and compression, interfering with the secretion of other tropic hormones. Other pituitary tumors may be associated with lactotroph hyperplasia and present with the characteristic syndrome of hyperprolactinemia and amenorrhea. With the utilization of the serum prolactin assay and the increased sensitivity of the new imaging techniques, the association of amenorrhea and small pituitary tumors has become recognized as a relatively common problem. This is not a new phenomenon, rather it reflects more sensitive diagnostic techniques. Attempts to link the problem to oral contraceptive use, have proved negative.[14]

8. Increased prolactin concentrations may result from nonpituitary sources such as lung and renal tumors, and even a uterine leiomyoma. Severe renal disease requiring hemodialysis is associated with elevated prolactin levels due to the decreased glomerular filtration rate.

Clinical Evaluation

Hyperprolactinemia may be associated with a variety of menstrual cycle disturbances, including oligoovulation, corpus luteum insufficiency, as well as amenorrhea. About one third of women with secondary amenorrhea will have elevated prolactin concentrations. Pathologic hyperprolactinemia inhibits the pulsatile secretion of GnRH, and the reduction of circulating prolactin levels restores menstrual function.

Not all patients with hyperprolactinemia display galactorrhea. The reported incidence is about 33%. The disparity may not be due entirely to the variable zeal for which the presence of nipple milk secretion is sought during physical examination. The absence of galactorrhea may be due to the usual accompanying hypoestrogenic state. A more attractive explanation focuses on the concept of heterogeneity of tropic hormones. The radioimmunoassay for prolactin may not discriminate between heterogeneous molecules of prolactin. A high circulating level of prolactin may not represent material capable of interacting with breast prolactin receptors. On the other hand, galactorrhea can be seen in women with normal prolactin serum concentrations. Episodic fluctuations and sleep increments may account for this clinical discordance, or, in this case, bioactive prolactin may be present which is immunoactively not detectable.

If galactorrhea has been present for 6 months to 1 year, or hyperprolactinemia is noted in the process of working up menstrual disturbances, infertility, or hirsutism, the probability of a pituitary tumor must be recognized. The initial evaluation includes measurement of thyroid stimulating hormone (TSH) and prolactin, and radiologic evaluation of the sella turcica with a lateral, coned-down view.

In recent years, the radiologic evaluation of the pituitary area has undergone rapid change. There now is no argument that magnetic resonance imaging (MRI) is the diagnostic modality of choice, but it is very expensive and requires a lengthy period of time to obtain the images. The CT scan is also very good, but it too is expensive. The intention of the workup should be to isolate those few patients who require the more sophisticated and expensive methods.

Because small tumors need not be treated at all, the initial x-ray evaluation should be the coned-down view of the sella turcica. Combining this screening technique with the prolactin assay, the few patients requiring the more expensive methods can be selected. If the prolactin level is greater than 100 ng/ml, or if the coned-down view is abnormal, we recommend the MRI. The presence of visual problems and/or headaches also requires the more sensitive radiologic evaluation.

With the current diagnostic techniques there is no difficulty in discovering and monitoring the size and function of a pituitary prolactin secreting tumor. With few exceptions the combination of elevation in basal levels of prolactin and radiographic imaging offers complete confidence in diagnosing sellar pathology. The major concern remains in determining management—medical, surgical, or expectant? The considerations that influence management include:

1. Microadenomas, if exclusively prolactin producing, rarely progress to macroadenoma size. Most are exceedingly slow growing or stable.
2. The histology of many so-called tumors is not one of neoplasia. Most contain nodular or diffuse hyperplasia of basically normal lactotrophs.
3. It is possible that a primary hypothalamic dysfunction which drives the lactotroph to hyperfunction and hyperplasia is the fundamental factor in the genesis of these "tumors." Thus, uncertain long-term cures, recurrence, and new tumor formation remain possibilities.
4. Some tumors regress spontaneously. Medical therapy (the dopamine agonist, bromocriptine) shrinks tumors and can prevent growth, although complete elimination of a tumor by bromocriptine does not occur, and rapid regrowth can follow discontinuation of bromocriptine treatment.
5. Transsphenoidal microsurgery is a very safe procedure, but there is a high recurrence rate.

Treatment of Galactorrhea

Galactorrhea as an isolated symptom of hypothalamic dysfunction existing in an otherwise healthy woman does not require treatment. Periodic prolactin levels will, if within the normal range, confirm the stability of the underlying process. However, some patients find the presence or amount of galactorrhea sexually, cosmetically, or emotionally burdensome. Bromocriptine is the drug of choice for treatment. Even with normal prolactin concentrations and a normal skull x-ray, treatment with bromocriptine can eliminate galactorrhea.

We have adopted a conservative approach of close surveillance for pituitary prolactin-secreting adenomas, recommending surgery only for those tumors that display rapid growth or those tumors that are already large and do not shrink in response to bromocriptine. If the prolactin level is greater than 100 ng/ml, or if the coned-down view of the sella turcica is abnormal, we recommend MRI. If MRI rules out an empty sella syndrome or a suprasellar problem, surgical intervention after preoperative bromocriptine treatment is then dictated by the patient's desires, the size of the tumor, and the response of the tumor to bromocriptine. Only on-going surveillance is necessary for patients with prolactin levels less than 100 ng/ml and with normal coned-down views of the sella turcica. An annual prolactin level and periodic coned-down views are indicated for continued observation to detect a growing tumor. Bromocriptine therapy is recommended for patients wishing to achieve pregnancy, and for those patients who have galactorrhea to the point of discomfort.

Headache

Headaches are very common, but it is rare when the cause of the headache is a serious problem. Most headaches are due to vasodilatation, muscle contraction, or psychologic stress. In order to avoid unnecessary investigation, therefore, it is important to identify the patient who warrants a more aggressive evaluation.

Vascular Headaches. Acute and throbbing headaches are due to abnormal vasodilatation. The vasodilatation associated with migraine headaches is believed to follow a period of vasoconstriction. Migraine headaches are usually, but not always, preceded by prodromal symptoms (which may reflect the period of vasoconstriction). Significant vascular headaches can be precipitated by stress, alcohol, or tyramine and tryptophan rich foods (red wine, chocolate, ripe cheeses). Vascular headaches can accompany other problems, such as systemic viral infections, fever, or hypertension.

Tension Headaches. The common tension headache is due to prolonged and excessive muscle contraction. The pain is dull, steady, bilateral, and worsens throughout the day.

Traction Headaches. This type of headache is due to pressure or pulling of structures. Headache associated with brain tumors are usually accompanied by neurologic abnormalities. Other causes are brain abscesses, subdural hematomas, and concussions.

Inflammatory Headaches. The main cause of inflammatory headaches is meningitis.

Evaluation

The acute onset of severe headache pain deserves attention. The following signs suggest the presence of a serious problem: neck stiffness, altered mental status, focal neurologic abnormalities, visual impairment, and fever. Any patient with meningeal signs requires hospitalization. Keep carbon monoxide exposure and drug withdrawal in mind as etiologic agents.

Chronic headaches should be characterized according to location, quality, and course over time. Head trauma in the past is an important piece of information, raising the suspicion of a subdural hematoma. When the headache is cyclic, with periodic complete resolution, one can comfortably ascribe the headache to a vascular origin. Tension headaches are either variable or relatively constant without relentless progression. Any recurrent or chronic headache that gets worse with time deserves a neurologic evaluation.

Management

Case-control studies with the old higher dose oral contraceptives indicated that migraine headaches were linked to a risk of stroke. Strokes are essentially no longer seen with low dose oral contraception. This probably reflects both lower dosage as well as the reluctance of clinicians to prescribe oral contraception to women with severe headaches.

The run of the mill headache is treated with mild analgesics such as aspirin, acetaminophen, or the nonsteroidal antiinflammatory agents. A problem of severe headaches on oral contraception requires an immediate response. The conservative reaction is to discontinue the oral contraceptives. On the other hand, the headache can be due to stress or some other reversible condition. We would argue that automatic discontinuation of oral contraception is not necessary with the low dose preparations. It would be better to evaluate the patient and find out if the patient can continue her contraceptive protection, by discovering an explanation for the headaches.

True severe vascular headaches are an indication to discontinue oral contraception. The symptom complex which deserves serious consideration includes: headaches which last a long time; dizziness, nausea, or vomiting with headaches; scotomata or blurred vision; episodes of blindness; unilateral, unremitting headaches; and headaches which continue despite medication.

In some women, a relationship exists between their fluctuating hormone levels during a menstrual cycle and migraine headaches, with the onset of headaches characteristically coinciding with menses. We have had personal success (anecdotal to be sure) alleviating headaches by eliminating the menstrual cycle, either with the use of *daily* oral contraceptives or the daily administration of a progestational agent (such as 10 mg medroxyprogesterone acetate). Some women with migraine headaches have extremely gratifying responses.

Concern over headaches with oral contraception should be limited to the use of combined oral contraceptives. The progestin-only methods are not associated with problems with headaches. Therefore, the sustained release progestin-only methods are also free of headache concern.

Uterine Fibroids

Uterine fibroids, more correctly referred to as leiomyomas, are benign tumors originating in the muscle cells of the uterus. Although the highest incidence occurs in women in their 50s, it is not uncommon to encounter these tumors during the reproductive years. Leiomyomas are more common in black women, usually multiple, and more likely to grow and become symptomatic in nulliparous women.

Leiomyomas which lie just beneath the endometrium, submucosal leiomyomas, cause the most trouble. Submucosal fibroids cause bleeding problems, and depending upon size and location, infertility and recurrent abortion.

Leiomyomas appear to be dependent upon hormone stimulation, specifically estrogen. Therefore, it is not surprising that they usually shrink after menopause. In the past, fibroids were known to grow in women using extremely high dose estrogen oral contraceptives. This is extremely rare, if it occurs at all, with the present low dose formulations. Long-term use of higher dose oral contraceptives was associated with a significantly reduced risk of developing fibroids.[15] It remains to be seen whether this benefit will persist with the current low dose formulations.

The majority of uterine fibroids can be easily diagnosed by pelvic examination. Uncertainty requires a pelvic ultrasound examination, especially to make sure the mass is not due to an ovarian tumor.

Management. Small uterine fibroids can be safely managed by periodic (every 3–6 months) pelvic examination. We believe that patients with small, unchanging uterine fibroids can be provided oral contraception. It would be prudent to avoid the use of an IUD; no experience is available regarding pregnancy rates and expulsion rates in women with uterine fibroids. There is no reason to avoid the progestin-only methods.

Surgery is indicated for women with symptomatic uterine fibroids or rapidly enlarging fibroids. Usually, surgery is recommended when uterine fibrids reach the size of a 12 week gestation, even if asymptomatic. This is because it is at this size that symptoms begin, pressure on vital structures is exerted, and surgery becomes more difficult. Malignant change to a leiomyosarcoma is very rare and usually occurs after menopause, but if the uterus undergoes rapid enlargement in a premenopausal woman, leiomyosarcoma must be suspected.

References

1. Larsen B, Galask RP, Vaginal microbial flora composition and influences of host physiology, Ann Intern Med 96:926, 1982.

2. Stein GE, Christensen S, Mummaw N, Comparative study of fluconazole and clotrimazole in the treatment of vulvovaginal candidiasis, DICP, Ann Pharmacotherap 25:582, 1991.

3. Sobel JD, Recurrent vulvovaginal candidiasis: a prospective study of the efficacy of maintenance ketoconzole therapy, New Engl J Med 315:1455, 1986.

4. Malouf M, Fortier M, Morin G, Dube JL, Treatment of Hemophilus vaginalis vaginitis, Obstet Gynecol 57:711, 1981.

5. McLellan R, Spence MR, Brockman M, Raffel L, Smith JL, The clinical diagnosis of trichomoniasis, Obstet Gynecol 60:30, 1982.

6. Krieger JN, Tam MR, Stevens CE, Nielsen IO, Hale J, Kiviat NB, Holmes KK, Diagnosis of trichomoniasis. Comparison of conventional wet mount examination with cytologic studies, cultures, and monoclonal antibody staining of direct specimens, JAMA 259:1223, 1988.

7. Schaeffer AJ, Recurrent urinary tract infections in women, Postgrad Med 81:51, 1987.

8. Pye JK, Mansel RE, Hughes LE, Clinical experience of drug treatments for mastalgia, Lancet ii:373, 1985.

9. Fentiman IS, Brame K, Caleffi M, Chaudary MA, Hayward JL, Double-blind controlled trial of tamoxifen therapy for mastalgia, Lancet i:287, 1986.

10. Ernster VL, Mason L, Goodson WH III, Sickles EA, Sacks ST, Selvin S, Dupuy ME, Hawkinson J, Hunt TK, Effects of caffeine-free diet on benign breast disease: A randomized trial, Surgery 91:263, 1982.

11. Lubin F, Ron E, Wax Y, Black M, Funaro M, Shitrit A, A case-control study of caffeine and methylxanthines in benign breast disease, JAMA 253:2388, 1985.

12. Schairer C, Brinton LA, Hoover RN, Methylxanthines and benign breast disease, Am J Epidemiol 124:603, 1986.

13. Hwang PLH, Ng CSA, Cheong ST, Effect of oral contraceptives on serum prolactin: A longitudinal study in 126 normal premenopausal women, Clin Endocrinol 24:127, 1986.

14. Pituitary Adenoma Study Group, Pituitary adenomas and oral contraceptives: a multicenter case-control study, Fertil Steril 39:753, 1983.

15. Ross RK, Pike MC, Vessey MP, Bull D, Yeates D, Casagrande JT, Risk factors for uterine fibroids: Reduced risk associated with oral contraceptives, Br J Med 293:359, 1986.

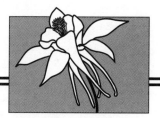

Epilogue

AND SO WE REACH our final paragraph. We do so with optimism. This book documents, within a tick of planet Earth's time, tremendous accomplishments in contraception. These accomplishments reflect initiative, creativity, and dedication. There is reason to believe, as we do, that these human traits will persevere, and we will meet the contraceptive challenges of the future.

Index